Introduction to
Health Care

Finance and Accounting

Introduction to
Health Care

Finance and Accounting

Carlene Harrison • William P. Harrison

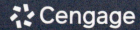

Australia • Brazil • Canada • Mexico • Singapore • United Kingdom • United States

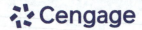

Introduction to Health Care Finance and Accounting, Second Edition

Carlene Harrison
William P. Harrison

SVP, Product: Erin Joyner

VP, Product: Thais Alencar

Portfolio Product Director: Jason Fremder

Portfolio Product Manager: Andrea Henderson

Product Assistant: Bridget Duffy

Learning Designer: Debra Myette-Flis

Content Manager: Amanda White

Digital Project Manager: Lisa Christopher

VP, Product Marketing: Jason Sakos

Director, Product Marketing: Neena Bali

Product Marketing Manager: Joann Gillingham

Content Acquisition Analyst: Erin McCullough

Production Service: Straive

Designer: Felicia Bennett

Cover Image Source: Felicia Bennett

Interior image Source: Pamela Johnston

For product information and technology assistance, contact us at
Cengage Customer & Sales Support, 1-800-354-9706
or support.cengage.com.

For permission to use material from this text or product, submit all requests online at **www.copyright.com**.

Library of Congress Control Number: 2023901420

ISBN-13: 978-0-357-62204-9

ISBN-10: 0-357-62204-9

Cengage
200 Pier 4 Boulevard
Boston, MA 02210
USA

Cengage is a leading provider of customized learning solutions. Our employees reside in nearly 40 different countries and serve digital learners in 165 countries around the world. Find your local representative at **www.cengage.com**.

To learn more about Cengage platforms and services, register or access your online learning solution, or purchase materials for your course, visit **www.cengage.com**.

Notice to the Reader

Printed in Mexico
Print Number: 1   Print Year: 2023

Contents

Chapter 3: The Rising Costs of Medical Services and Health Care Reform.. 39

Section II:
Accounting For Healthcare Facilities   59

Section III: Health Care Financial Management   129

About the Authors

Carlene Harrison, Ed.D., was Dean of the School of Allied Health at Hodges University. As dean, her overall responsibility was for four degree programs: Health Administration, Health Studies, Medical Assisting, and Health Information Management. Before becoming a full-time educator, she was an administrator in several outpatient healthcare facilities for over 20 years, including for-profit, not-for-profit, and public health organizations. Her doctorate is from Argosy University. Her dissertation research looked at improvement in critical thinking in adult learners. She is the author of three other healthcare-related textbooks.

William P. Harrison, M.B.A., retired from a career in public finance spanning four decades. Working with public agencies, his areas of expertise included budgeting, investments, and accessing bond markets for capital financing. His areas of specialization also included development and monitoring of self-funded employee health insurance programs and implementation of protected self-insurance initiatives. He has a bachelor's degree in economics and a master of business administration degree in finance and accounting.

Contributing Author

Carol Taylor, MFT, MHRM, MPH and FJD Health Law, is the Health Care Management Program Director at Ultimate Medical Academy. As a Program Director, she is responsible for ensuring her students have the essential accounting skills necessary to prepare them for a healthcare career. She has healthcare experience working in hospital surgical units, human resources, dental organizations, and mental health treatment facilities. She has been an adjunct instructor for Kaplan University and Purdue University Global for more than 16 years, motivating students to achieve their career goals.

Acknowledgements

The contributing author would like to thank Dr. Elan Salee, owner of Boynton Dental Studio, for contributing photos of electronic medical devices and office photos to use in the textbook.

In addition, Cengage Learning Designer, Debra Myette Flis, who participated in several meetings reviewing content and making recommendations to ensure that we created a great learning experience for students.

Reviewers

Cengage would like to acknowledge and thank the following instructors for their feedback and suggestions for the second edition of *Introduction to Healthcare Finance and Accounting*.

Angela A. Gomez, DBA, Macc, MBA

Director of Accounting Programs, Latin Division; Professor
Keiser University, Online Division
Longwood, FL

Kaitlyn E. Junk, MBA, RRT-NPS

Instructor
Western Technical College
La Crosse, WI

Carol Taylor, MFT, MHRM, MPH & EJD Health Law

Program Director, Healthcare Management Program
Ultimate Medical Academy
Land O Lakes, FL

Joanne Muniz, DBA, CFE

Assistant Professor, Accounting
Webber International University
Babson Park, FL

Amelia Grayson

Professor
Seattle Central College
Fife, WA

Overview of the American Healthcare System

Financial management in health care comes with a unique set of challenges. Section I analyzes the differences between health care and other types of businesses and reviews the varied legal structures and missions of healthcare organizations. The evolution to third-party payers for healthcare services is traced from the start of healthcare insurance to government involvement in financing health care. The issues of rising medical costs and the impacts of the Patient Protection and Affordable Care Act of 2010 (PPACA) bring healthcare financial management to the present day.

The Environment of Healthcare Finance

Key Terms

Capitation plans
Certificate of Need (CON)
Corporation
Equity
Fee-for-service
Health maintenance organizations (HMOs)
Hospice care
Hospital Survey and Construction Act of 1946
Inpatient facilities
Limited liability partnership (LLP)
Long-term-care facilities
Managed care
Outpatient facilities
Palliative care
Partnership
Preferred provider
Professional corporation (PC)
Professional association (PA)
Proprietorship
Spend-down
Tax Equity and Fiscal Responsibility Act of 1982 (TEFRA)
Telehealth services

Chapter Objectives

After completing this chapter, readers should be able to:

- Explain the similarities and differences of health care from other types of businesses.

- Discuss the background of financing health care in the United States.

- Analyze the factors causing the growth of inpatient hospital facilities until the mid-1980s and the decline after that time.

- Identify the variety of services provided in outpatient settings.

- Analyze the growth in outpatient services and home-based services.

- Describe the functions of nursing homes, the rise of life-care facilities, and hospice care as a specialty within health care.

- Describe the legal differences between proprietorships, partnerships, and corporations.

- Explain the use of professional corporations (PCs) and limited liability partnerships (LLPs) to control business liability.

- Discuss the differences in function and mission between for-profit, not-for-profit, and governmental healthcare organizations.

BOX 1-1 Types of Medical Businesses

1. For-profit healthcare organizations
- Proprietorships and professional corporations (PCs)
- Partnerships and limited liability partnerships (LLPs)
- Small corporations
- Large publicly held corporations

2. Not-for-profit business-style organizations

3. Government healthcare facilities

4. Other healthcare organizations

For-Profit Healthcare Organizations: Proprietorships and Professional Corporations (PCs)

A **proprietorship**, also referred to as a **sole proprietorship**, is a business owned by one individual. Proprietorships are easy to form, not requiring the legal documentation of partnership agreements or corporate charters. When a proprietorship business has a profit, evidenced by annual revenues in excess of annual expenses, the profit is taxed as income to the owner whether it is reinvested in the business or withdrawn from the business by the owner in the form of a salary.

Example 1-1

Dr. Tompkins attended the University of Michigan Medical School and had her postgraduate training at a major Detroit hospital. In 2000, she started a private practice in her hometown in rural Michigan. She hired an office manager who also served as bookkeeper and two medical assistants to assist in the practice. Dr. Tompkins uses a local accountant to prepare financial statements and tax returns as a sole proprietorship.

Proprietorships have several major disadvantages. The business owner, wishing to recover their investment in the business, will not find an organized market that may be easily accessed for selling the business. A physician wishing to retire from private practice may face a lengthy process in attracting a new physician to purchase the practice and structuring the sale. This is different from an individual holding stock in a hospital corporation listed on a major stock exchange. In that case, the stock may be easily sold and the equity position converted to cash.

A second major disadvantage is that the owner of a proprietorship has unlimited personal liability for any debts or legal settlements against the business. If the business loses money and is closed with debts still outstanding, creditors have the ability to collect funds due them from the personal assets of the owner. To address this issue of unlimited liability, all 50 states have statutes that allow proprietorships to form a **professional corporation (PC)**. In some states, this is referred to as a **professional association (PA)**. While providing protections to the business owner, professional liability for malpractice is not covered and remains the responsibility of the individual physician.

Partnerships and Limited Liability Partnerships (LLPs)

A **partnership** is a business owned by two or more individuals or entities. Partnerships in health care are most commonly two or more individual medical professionals in business together to provide services. As in a proprietorship, profits generated by the business are taxed as income to the partners. Profits are divided by the partners based on the partnership agreement that can range from a simple oral agreement to a complex written document.

Example 1-2

Dr. Tompkins, from Example 1-1, opened her practice in 2000. Over the years, her hometown has grown and her practice with it. In 2008, Dr. Tompkins hired Dr. Restin to a salaried position with no equity position in the practice. The term equity represents an ownership position in a business. In 2011, Dr. Tompkins contacted a local attorney and had him prepare a partnership agreement for the practice, making Dr. Restin an equal partner. The business is now a legal partnership between the two physicians.

Partnerships have the same disadvantages as proprietorships, including a limited market for the sale of partnership equity and in the unlimited liability of the partners. This issue of unlimited liability has been addressed by legislation to provide financial protection to partners in a medical business. **Limited liability partnerships (LLPs)** are available under a number of state statutes. These LLPs retain unlimited liability to the partners for most debts, but any debts resulting from malpractice settlements are the responsibility of the individual physician responsible for the malpractice, not the partners. The legal structure of a PC, discussed earlier in the section on proprietorships, is also available to a medical partnership.

Comprehension Check 1.2

In the following questions, identify if the type of medical business is a proprietorship, partnership, or an LLP.

1. Dr. Evans was working for a major dental organization after completing his externship and passing the Dental National Board Examination, Florida Laws and Rules Examination, and ADEX Dental Licensing Examination. Dr. Evans decided to gain experience while working for a major dental organization for several years. Dr. Evans opened his own dental practice. Dr. Evans hired two dental assistants, a hygienist and an office manager. What type of medical business would this be?

2. In January 2022, Dr. Evans and Dr. Briggs noticed an increase in business within the dental practice that they have formed as a partnership. They both decide to form a partnership where they will both be individually responsible for any malpractice settlements. What type of medical business would this be?

3. Dr. Evans' business has doubled within the last two years. More staff have been hired. There are now two additional dental assistants, one additional dental hygienist, and a biller and coder. In January 2021, Dr. Evans hires Dr. Briggs and decides to make her an equal partner. An agreement is signed between Dr. Evans and Dr. Briggs. What type of medical business would this be?

Small For-Profit Corporations

Any business can be organized as a corporation, requiring only a corporate charter and a set of bylaws. Corporations may be privately held or owned by a single person or a small group of people. In a privately or closely held corporation, the owners are private investors. Small corporations may function in a fashion very similar to a proprietorship or partnership, with no market for the capital stock and the future of the business dependent on the work of the owner or partners. Small corporations, with stock held by a single individual or just a few stockholders, may be incorporated as **S corporations** under the Internal Revenue Code. In these S corporations, profits of the corporation are passed through to the stockholders and taxed as income.

Large Publicly Held Corporations

Publicly held corporations raise funds by issuing stock. Many of these large corporations have thousands of stockholders, and the stock of these companies is actively traded on major stock markets. In the world of business, think of General Electric and Microsoft. In medical services, these large investor-owned businesses include Health Management Associates (HMA) and Tenet Healthcare Corporation in hospital management, Walgreens and CVS in pharmacies, healthcare insurance companies such as United Healthcare, and large corporations doing business in nursing homes and life-care facilities (LCFs). These large corporations will continue to provide their goods and services indefinitely, surviving the death or departure of key executives and individual stockholders.

Example 1-3

Tenet Healthcare Corporation is an example of a large publicly held corporation in health care. On Tenet's website (www.tenethealth.com), they report that they own and operate 49 hospitals in 11 states and 63 outpatient facilities in 12 states. A Standard & Poor's stock report stated in April 2011 that Tenet had 2010 total revenues of $9.2 billion. The corporation had 846 million shares of capital stock outstanding and a total market value of $3.4 billion.

One of the major advantages of the corporate structure is that the corporation has an unlimited life, not limited to the lifespan of the owner or partners. A second major advantage to the corporation is that it is a separate and distinct legal entity and the liability of the stockholders is limited to the value of the investment made in the stock. Under this concept of limited liability, if the company becomes bankrupt, debts owed by the business are paid up to the limits of the assets held by the corporation and creditors are precluded from making claims against the stockholders.

Example 1-4

To illustrate the concept of limited liability: GenX Biotech is a new research company that has a public stock offering. Tom Adams, an individual investor, purchases $5,000 of GenX Biotech stock at the initial public offering. Capital raised from the stock offering is supplemented with a bank line of credit. The company conducts basic research in hopes of developing marketable products. After three years, the company has exhausted all its resources and fails. The stock purchased by Mr. Adams is now worthless, but he is not personally responsible for any of the debts of the company.

One of the major trends in U.S. medicine over the past several decades has been the rise of for-profit hospital corporations purchasing and managing a number of hospitals. Centralized functions such as administration, corporate accounting, and purchasing can lead to cost-efficiencies and greater profits. Large for-profit systems may own hundreds of hospitals across the country. Public stock offerings and cash generated by operations provide funding for further acquisitions and generating value for stockholders. Management and corporate planning will be centered within corporate headquarters, with the day-to-day operations of individual hospitals handled locally.

The major financial disadvantage for large publicly held corporations is double taxation. Businesses with a standard corporate structure are referred to as **C corporations** in the federal tax code. These corporations are required to pay taxes on profits made in their business activities. Then when the profits are distributed to stockholders in the form of dividends, they are taxed again as income on individual tax reports.

Not-For-Profit Business Organizations

Many communities are served by not-for-profit hospitals. These hospitals operate in a business style similar to for-profit hospitals, with the revenues received from providing medical services used to cover their costs of operation. Where a for-profit business **may** decide to adopt a corporate structure, not-for-profit businesses (also called nonprofits) **must** be structured as corporations. For-profit businesses are established and operated to make money and share the profits with stockholders in the form of dividends and growth in the value of the stock. Not-for-profits provide for the public good and are not designed to earn profits. Businesses that meet the qualifications as not-for-profit are exempt from both property and income taxes under Internal Revenue Code Section 501(c)(3) as charitable organizations. That section provides the following definition of a charitable organization: "any corporation, community chest, fund, or foundation that is organized and operated exclusively for religious, charitable, scientific, public safety, literary, or educational purposes."

A for-profit business has stockholders who elect a board of directors to oversee the operations of the entity. A not-for-profit corporation has an appointed board, generally comprising community leaders dedicated to the charitable mission of the entity. However, there are no stockholders to whom the board is accountable.

Comprehension Check 1.3

1. Dr. Harden just graduated from veterinary medicine school. With the increase of animal abandonment, she decided to open a shelter for misplaced animals. Her focus is to educate the public on resources within the community to lessen animal abandonment rates. Through researching how to establish her shelter, she discovered that under the Internal Revenue Code Section 501(c)(3) her shelter would fall under a charitable organization. Is Dr. Harden operating a profit or nonprofit business?

One of the areas of uniqueness in the healthcare industry comes from the competition of a for-profit entity and a not-for-profit entity in the same marketplace. For-profit hospitals are outnumbered by nongovernment, not-for-profit hospitals. It is not uncommon for a large community to be served by both for-profit hospitals and not-for-profit hospitals. Not-for-profit hospitals have the advantages of not having to generate profits for stockholders and frequently enjoy community donor and volunteer support. For-profit hospitals that are part of multihospital holding companies have available cost savings from the centralization of functions such as purchasing and accounting to hold down operating costs.

Government Healthcare Facilities

Federal, state, and local units of government are heavily involved in directly providing medical services. The U.S. Department of Veterans Affairs (VA) owns and operates medical facilities nationwide, providing services to veterans and their families. In many communities, local governments own hospitals that are operated as a service to the citizens. In low-income areas, these government-run hospitals are able to support operating revenues with local taxes to be able to continue services. County health departments provide services to the communities, supported by local taxes.

Other Healthcare Organizations

A number of healthcare organizations that provide medical services directly to patients and clients do not fit neatly into the previous business categories. These are primarily voluntary health and welfare organizations that rely on public donations for their funding. Examples of these types of organizations would be the American Red Cross, the March of Dimes, and Planned Parenthood.

Table 1-1 shows the number of community, nonprofit, profit, government, and other hospitals in the United States.

Table 1-1: Total Number of all U.S. Hospitals

Total Number of All U.S. Hospitals	6,090
Number of U.S. **Community**[1] Hospitals	5,141
Number of Nongovernment Not-for-Profit Community Hospitals	2,946
Number of Investor-Owned (For-Profit) Community Hospitals	1,233
Number of State and Local Government Community Hospitals	962
Number of Federal Government Hospitals	208
Number of Nonfederal Psychiatric Hospitals	625
Other[2] Hospitals	116

[1] **Community hospitals** are defined as all nonfederal, short-term general, and other special hospitals. Community hospitals include academic medical centers or other teaching hospitals if they are nonfederal short-term hospitals. Excluded are hospitals not accessible by the general public, such as prison hospitals or college infirmaries.

[2] **Other hospitals** include nonfederal long-term-care hospitals and hospital units within an institution such as a prison hospital or school infirmary. Long-term-care hospitals may be defined by different methods; here they include other hospitals with an average length of stay of 30 or more days.

Source: From AHA site. https://www.aha.org/statistics/fast-facts-us-hospitals

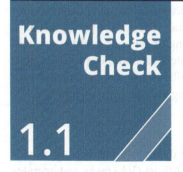

Knowledge Check 1.1

1. What are the major differences between financial management for healthcare facilities and other types of free-enterprise businesses?

_____

_____

_____

continued

2. What types of skills do you think are necessary for an effective financial manager in health care?

_____

_____

_____

3. Dr. Reginald Dustin is a licensed family practice physician. He has hired a staff of five to help him in running the practice. He draws a monthly salary and leaves profits in the business for capital purchases. This type of business is a:

A. Proprietorship

B. Partnership

C. For-profit corporation

D. Not-for-profit corporation

4. Dr. Towers has an established medical practice and wishes to expand the practice by bringing in another physician. The two physicians agree to a document specifying how much the new physician will pay into the business over time to secure an equity position, their monthly salary draws, and a division of profits. This type of business is a:

A. Proprietorship

B. Partnership

C. For-profit corporation

D. Not-for-profit corporation

5. American Hospitals owns and operates 18 hospitals in 11 states. It is registered with the Securities & Exchange Commission and has several thousand stockholders. This type of business is a:

A. Proprietorship

B. Partnership

C. For-profit corporation

D. Not-for-profit corporation

6. What is a professional corporation (PC), and why would this structure be an advantage to a physician?

_____

_____

_____

7. What is a 501(c)(3) corporation?

_____

_____

_____

_____

Table 1-3: Telehealth Services Increased During 2020

	February		April		
	Total Primary Care Visits	**Percent Telehealth**	**Total Primary Care Visits**	**Percent Telehealth**	**Medicare COVID-19 Hospitalizations per Thousand Beneficiaries**
US Total	**19,655,604**	**0.1%**	**4,786,049**	**43.5%**	**11.7**
Boston, NA	355,687	0.0%	237,694	73.1%	35.7
Minneapolis-St. Paul, MN	123,001	0.1%	71,806	63.9%	4.9
Philadelphia, PA	416,398	0.0%	229,355	61.6%	24.0
San Francisco, CA	187,845	0.2%	105,112	60.2%	3.7
Detroit, MI	225,850	0.1%	126,331	59.7%	60.3
New York, NY	1,233,990	0.1%	634,558	56.5%	59.5
Chicago, IL	512,752	0.0%	289,301	52.4%	24.5
Dallas, TX	320,465	0.0%	188,693	52.2%	4.8
Washington, DC	372,015	0.1%	209,979	50.7%	12.8
Seattle, WA	159,261	0.1%	84,928	48.2%	7.5
Los Angeles, CA	529,503	0.1%	300,283	46.3%	16.3
Houston, TX	257,008	0.0%	144,313	46.2%	7.1
Miami, FL	366,302	0.0%	198,779	43.9%	21.3
Atlanta, GA	260,596	0.0%	138,613	42.1%	10.5
Phoenix, AZ	315,174	0.0%	185,470	37.8%	4.2

Note: Hospitalization rates calculated using Medicare claims among Inpatient Prospective Payment System (IPPS)/Critical Access Hospitals (CAH) hospitals. Rates reported as 0 percent may include some hospitalizations but are below 0.1 percent.

Source: https://aspe.hhs.gov/reports/medicare-beneficiary-use-telehealth-visits-early-data-start-covid-19-pandemic

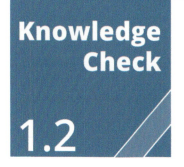

Knowledge Check

1.2

1. Describe the impact of the Tax Equity and Fiscal Responsibility Act of 1982 (TEFRA) on hospital finances.

_____

_____

_____

continued

2. What is the major difference between a general hospital and a specialty hospital? Provide examples of specialty hospitals.

_____

_____

_____

3. What has been the financial impact on hospitals of the decline in inpatient care over the past 25 years?

_____

_____

_____

4. Which of the following would not be considered an outpatient facility?
A. A physician's family care office practice
B. A walk-in clinic
C. A dental surgery office
D. A rehabilitation hospital that provides short-term stays for recovery and rehabilitation treatments
E. All of the above are outpatient facilities.

5. What are the basic services provided by home healthcare organizations?

_____

_____

_____

6. Describe the physical and service changes in the transition from traditional nursing homes to modern model of life-care facilities (LCFs).

_____

_____

_____

7. How does hospice care differ from traditional medical care?

_____

_____

_____

8. Define palliative care.

_____

_____

_____

Key Concepts

- Financial management in health care shares many of the basic functions with other types of business but comes with its own unique set of circumstances and requirements.

- A proprietorship is a business owned by a single individual; in health care, it is most commonly found as the legal structure for physician practices.

- A partnership is a business entity owned by two or more individuals or entities.

- A for-profit corporation is a legal structure designed to have an unlimited life. Publicly held for-profit corporations have stockholders and are established to return value to the stockholders.

- A not-for-profit corporation is structured with a board of trustees and is designed to provide for the public good.

- Medical services provided in an inpatient setting peaked in the mid-1980s and have been declining with the expansion of outpatient services.

- Outpatient services, those not requiring an overnight stay, provide ambulatory and primary care to patients in a wide variety of specialties.

- Home-based medical services have expanded from a combination of a lower cost of providing services and patient preference for treatment in familiar surroundings.

- The scope of services provided in traditional nursing homes has expanded into the current model of LCFs, meeting the needs of residents throughout the later stages of life.

- Hospice care is a specialty in medicine, providing medical and emotional services to the patient and family members in the patient's last months of life.

Paying for Health Care

Chapter Objectives

After completing this chapter, readers should be able to:

- Compare and contrast fee-for-service and managed care private-sector healthcare insurance plans.

- Discuss the protections available to employees and their families in the Consolidated Omnibus Budget Reconciliation Act (COBRA).

- Explain the major public-policy issues in government healthcare programs available through Medicare and Medicaid.

- Identify the healthcare benefits available to members of the armed forces and their families.

- Describe the financial impact of the uninsured on the healthcare system in America.

used over the participant's lifetime. HDHP have been well received by healthy younger individuals and couples without dependents as a mechanism to build up funds for future medical expenses. The percentage of covered workers in HDHP rose from 8 percent of participants in healthcare insurance programs in 2009 to 13 percent in 2010. Table 2-1 shows the rates for an HDHP in 2022.

Table 2-1 High Deductible Health Plan Rates in 2022

	Minimum deductible (The amount you pay for healthcare items and services before your plan starts to pay)	Maximum out-of-pocket costs (The most you'd have to pay if you need more healthcare items and services)
Individual HDHP	$1,400	$7,050
Family HDHP	$2,800	$14,100

Knowledge Check

2.1

1. Discuss preferred provider organization (PPO) plans. What are the main advantages and disadvantages?

_____

_____

_____

2. Discuss health maintenance organizations (HMOs). What are the main advantages and disadvantages?

_____

_____

_____

Government Regulation of Private-Sector Healthcare Plans: Consolidated Omnibus Budget Reconciliation Act (COBRA)

"The Consolidated Omnibus Budget Reconciliation Act (COBRA) gives workers and their families who lose their health benefits the right to choose to continue group health benefits provided by their group health plan for limited periods of time under certain circumstances such as voluntary or involuntary job loss, reduction in hours worked, transition between jobs, death, divorce, and other life events."

(U.S. Department of Labor, www.dol.gov/dol/topic/.../cobra.htm)

Congress passed the **Consolidated Omnibus Budget Reconciliation Act (COBRA)** in 1986, providing former employees and their dependents the opportunity to continue group health insurance benefits with the former employer. Prior to COBRA, the threat of loss of healthcare insurance served as a barrier to the free movement of employees in advancing their careers. This was especially true for employees with family health issues. Employers commonly mandate a 30- to 90-day waiting period for new employees to be eligible for employer-sponsored healthcare insurance programs. An employee taking a new job could face several months without healthcare insurance.

The law generally applies to group health plans provided by employers with 20 or more employees. From the date of the change in status that triggers COBRA provisions, the employee or dependents have 60 days to elect to continue health plan coverage and are required to pay the full cost of the health insurance premiums at the group health insurance rates. COBRA coverage benefits covering individuals at group health insurance rates, even with the requirement of paying the full cost, will be a lower cost than paying the premiums for individual health coverage in the marketplace. Cost continues to be the principal downside to COBRA. The former employee electing to continue coverage under COBRA must pay the full cost of the insurance plus a modest fee for plan administration. Monthly premiums will be in the range of $300 to $500 for employee-only coverage and in excess of $1,000 monthly for family coverage. These costs make COBRA unaffordable for many former employees.

Qualifying events and time limits under COBRA are:

- When an employee is terminated, either voluntarily or involuntarily (for any reason other than "gross misconduct"), or has been reduced in hours worked, the employee, spouse, and dependent child(ren) are entitled to 18 months of continued coverage in the group health plan.

- When an employee reaches the age of 65 and is entitled to Medicare coverage, the spouse and dependent child(ren) may continue in the group health plan for up to 36 months.

- On the event of employee death, divorce, or legal separation, the spouse and dependent child(ren) may continue in the group health plan for up to 36 months.

- When a dependent child loses the status as dependent child, that individual may continue on the health plan for up to 36 months.

Table 2-2 shows the qualifying events, beneficiaries, and the maximum period of coverage.

Table 2-2 Maximum Period of Coverage Based on Qualifying Event

QUALIFYING EVENT	QUALIFIED BENEFICIARIES	MAXIMUM PERIOD OF CONTINUATION COVERAGE
Termination (for reasons other than gross misconduct) or reduction in hours of employment	Employee Spouse Dependent Child	18 months[2]
Employee enrollment in Medicare	Spouse Dependent Child	36 months[3]
Divorce or legal separation	Spouse Dependent Child	36 months
Death of employee	Spouse Dependent Child	36 months
Loss of "dependent child" status under the plan	Dependent Child	36 months

[2] In certain circumstances, qualified beneficiaries entitled to 18 months of continuation coverage may become entitled to a disability extension of an additional 11 months (for a total maximum of 29 months) or an extension of an additional 18 months due to the occurrence of a second qualifying event (for a total maximum of 36 months).

[3] The actual period of continuation coverage may vary depending on factors such as whether the Medicare entitlement occurred prior to or after the end of the covered employee's employment or reduction in hours. For more information, contact the Department of Labor's Employee Benefits Security Administration **electronically** or call toll free at **1-866-444-3272.**

Source: https://www.dol.gov/agencies/ebsa/laws-and-regulations/laws/cobra

COBRA benefits were amended and improved in the *American Recovery and Reinvestment Act of 2009 (ARRA)*, commonly referred to as the Stimulus Bill. Provisions in that law provided for a 65 percent premium subsidy to be paid to workers involuntarily terminated from their jobs. For the many Americans who lost their jobs due to the recession, paying $400 monthly for single healthcare coverage or $1,200 monthly for family coverage was not financially feasible. Many were forced to refuse COBRA coverage and joined the ranks of the uninsured. ARRA, with a 65 percent COBRA subsidy, allowed laid-off workers to continue healthcare coverage.

The original amendment provided this subsidy only for a period of nine months. It has since been extended by both the *Department of Defense Appropriations Act of 2010* and the *Continuing Extension Act of 2010.* These extensions allowed laid-off workers to continue healthcare insurance for themselves and their families at an affordable price.

Knowledge Check
2.2

1. John Miller is a 62-year-old X-ray technologist at a company with 50 employees who carries health insurance coverage for himself and his family through a plan sponsored by his employer. John elects to take early retirement. Can he continue to keep health insurance coverage through his former employer?

_____

_____

_____

2. In 2007, Susan Montgomery resigns her position as an HR coordinator for a healthcare facility to accept the position as controller for a local hospital. She was four months pregnant at the time of the change in jobs, and the hospital at that time had a preexisting clause in their health plan that would not cover the pregnancy. Can she continue to keep health insurance coverage through her former employer?

_____

_____

_____

3. Joe Sullivan is self-employed as a medical biller and coder who is covered by the health plan of his wife's employer, a major national retail chain. When Joe and his wife divorce, can he continue to keep health insurance coverage through his former wife's employer?

_____

_____

_____

4. Patricia Jeffries is employed at a small veterinary hospital with 12 employees. The hospital downsizes in the recession, and her job is eliminated. Can she continue to keep health insurance coverage through her former employer?

_____

_____

_____

Government Healthcare Programs

Any discussion of healthcare insurance in America cannot ignore the realities of the political landscape. Over the course of the twentieth and early twenty-first centuries, there has been almost continuous debate on the appropriate role of the federal government in financing health care as part of the broader discussion of "entitlements." Among elected officials, there have been a wide range of political views, making it difficult to reach consensus. Some have endorsed bringing healthcare insurance to the millions of American families not covered by employer-sponsored group health plans as a legitimate function of the federal government. Others have argued against what they consider to be unwarranted intrusion into what should be a private sector function and have raised concerns over program funding. Regardless of the merits of the two positions, the federal government is now deeply involved in health care.

Figure 2-2 shows how the federal budget is distributed toward defense, Social Security, and other health programs.

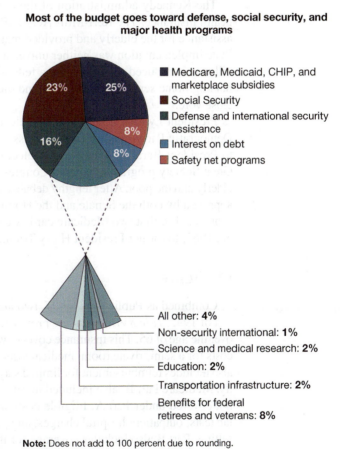

Most of the budget goes toward defense, social security, and major health programs

- 25% / 23% / 16% / 8% / 8%
- ■ Medicare, Medicaid, CHIP, and marketplace subsidies
- ■ Social Security
- ■ Defense and international security assistance
- ■ Interest on debt
- ■ Safety net programs

- All other: **4%**
- Non-security international: **1%**
- Science and medical research: **2%**
- Education: **2%**
- Transportation infrastructure: **2%**
- Benefits for federal retirees and veterans: **8%**

Note: Does not add to 100 percent due to rounding.

Figure 2-2 Where the Federal Budget Dollars Go

Source: 2019 figures from Office of Management and Budget, FY 2021 Historical Tables.

Expenditures by the federal government for healthcare costs are not limited to the 23 percent of the budget for the direct costs of Medicare and Medicaid. Other areas of the federal budget include costs for health care for current and retired federal employees, current and retired members of the armed forces, and specialized federal programs such as the Centers for Disease Control (CDC).

Social Security Amendments of 1965

Medicare, providing healthcare benefits to those generally over age 65, and Medicaid, a companion program establishing government reimbursement for healthcare costs for the indigent, were authorized in the Social Security Amendments of 1965. While 1965 witnessed the creation of these two programs, debate over a national program for healthcare insurance started 50 years earlier.

In 1915, labor groups made a failed attempt to introduce legislation in several states supporting national healthcare insurance. The Social Security Act of 1935 was approved into law as part of President Franklin D. Roosevelt's New Deal. This act provides retirement income to older Americans and is based on pay-as-you-go funding from payroll deductions on workers. President Roosevelt wanted to see health insurance coverage provided in addition to retirement income, but this potential expansion of the scope of the act was seen to be too controversial and was left out of the final legislation. The New Deal was followed by President Harry S. Truman's Fair Deal. The Fair Deal again raised the issue of national health insurance but limited the scope of the proposed program to the elderly. President Truman was not able to move this program forward but did serve to keep the debate over national health insurance alive.

The Kennedy administration of the early 1960s again raised the issue of national health insurance. The Kerr-Mills Act of 1960 authorized the states to establish medical assistance for the elderly and provided matching federal funds for these state programs. State implementation was neither universal nor consistent. In 1962, the King-Anderson bill was introduced to provide for a federal program covering the costs of hospital and nursing home services for those 65 and older. The bill was defeated in committee on a close vote.

President Lyndon B. Johnson was elected in 1964 and came into office enjoying a Democratic Party majority in Congress, the identical set of circumstances presented to President Barack Obama on his election in 2008. President Johnson outlined his Great Society program and urged Congress to address national health insurance for the elderly and the poor. After lengthy debate and compromise, Medicare and Medicaid were approved by both the Senate and the House of Representatives and signed by President Johnson. The first two Medicare cards were presented at the signing ceremony on July 30, 1965, to former President Harry Truman and his wife, Bess.

Medicare

Combined as Public Law 89-97, two amendments were made to the Social Security Act of 1935. *Title XVIII Medicare* provided Part A, covering hospital insurance for those over the age of 65. This insurance covers overnight inpatient hospital stays, including the costs for a semiprivate room, medical tests, and other appropriate inpatient costs. Part A also includes reimbursement for limited stays for convalescence in a skilled nursing facility. Medicare Part B, also included in Title XVIII, provides medical insurance for costs not covered under Part A. Eligible costs include the outpatient costs for doctor visits, lab tests, outpatient hospital charges, and physician services performed in an outpatient setting. Part B also includes coverage for the costs of durable medical equipment, such as wheelchairs and prosthetic devices.

The costs of the Medicare program are partially funded by working Americans who are assessed a 1.45 percent payroll tax, matched by the employer. Self-employed individuals are taxed at the rate of 2.9 percent of their annual net income. Unlike the 6.2 percent payroll tax for Social Security (reduced to 4.2 percent for 2011 and 2012 as a federal economic initiative to stimulate the economy), there is no upper limit to Medicare tax contributions. Since the implementation of Medicare in 1965, medical care costs have exceeded the rate of cost increases in the overall economy, requiring financial support from general revenues to support the programs. Payroll taxes support approximately 85 percent of Medicare Part A, hospitalization. For Medicare Part B, beneficiary premiums pay for only around one-quarter of program expenditures, the balance funded by general revenues of the government and contributing to the federal deficit. As of 2010, 47 million Americans were enrolled in the Medicare program.

Balanced Budget Act of 1997

The first major change to Medicare came with the passage of the **Balanced Budget Act of 1997**. Up to that time, Medicare was strictly a government-run program, paying standardized medical benefits under Part A and Part B to providers. In 1997, Medicare Part C was authorized, creating Medicare Advantage (MA) plans, providing eligible recipients of Medicare with the opportunity to receive their benefits from a number of private health insurance plans. MA plans are required to provide benefits equal to or greater than the standard Medicare and frequently provide extra benefits such as dental and vision insurance for a premium charge that is in addition to the standard Medicare Part B premium. Seniors are allowed to choose a plan that best meets their needs and budget and agree to use providers of medical services approved in the plan. MA plans operate in a similar fashion to the managed care provided by HMOs, with Medicare paying the plan a monthly capitated rate.

Medicare Prescription Drug, Improvement, and Modernization Act of 2003 (MMA)

In 2003, Congress closed a major gap in health insurance coverage for senior citizens with the passage of **Medicare Prescription Drug, Improvement, and Modernization Act of 2003 (MMA)**. The act authorized prescription drug coverage for all individuals either eligible for benefits under Medicare Part A or enrolled in Medicare Part B. Those entitled to drug coverage benefits are able to access the plan either through a Prescription Drug Plan (PDP) for standalone drug coverage or join an MA plan that combines medical service coverage with drug coverage.

Final details of the act, in a process common to all healthcare legislation, were the subject of debate and compromise, which ended up with the infamous "donut hole" in coverage. For 2010, individuals in the plan were covered for up to $2,830 in prescription drug costs after a deductible and coinsurance. After that amount had been reached, individuals were required to pay for their drugs up to a total out-of-pocket amount of $4,550, when the plan again began paying for what are referred to as "catastrophic costs." The financial cost to seniors caught in the donut hole who were required to pay for the costs of prescriptions after the $2,830 plan coverage was met has been addressed in the 2010 healthcare legislation. A combination of discounts on both brand name and generic drugs and phased reductions in the threshold for catastrophic coverage eliminated the gap between them in 2020.

Premium payments from beneficiaries provide only about 10 percent of the revenues to support the PDP. The balance of funding comes from general revenues.

In a 2011 report, the Congressional Budget Office (CBO) forecasted 2010 Medicare expenditures at $528 billion, a significant contributor to the estimated federal deficit of $1.3 trillion for the year. The report projected that Medicare expenditures will almost double by 2020, to $1.038 trillion. The report, titled *The Budget and Economic Outlook: Fiscal Years 2010 to 2020*, concluded: "To keep annual deficits and total federal debt from reaching levels that would substantially harm the economy, lawmakers would have to increase revenues significantly as a percentage of GDP, decrease projected spending sharply, or enact some combination of the two."

The CBO projects that, under current law, federal spending on Medicare and Medicaid measured as a share of GDP will rise from 4 percent today to 12 percent in 2050 and 19 percent in 2082—which, as a share of the economy, is roughly equivalent to the total amount that the federal government spends today.

Medicaid

Title XIX, Medicaid, established a new entitlement program that required each state to establish and fund healthcare security programs for those individuals at or near the public assistance level. Where Medicare eligibility is based on age, Medicaid eligibility is based on income. The federal government sets minimum eligibility and coverage standards and allows states to provide additional benefits. Federal funding to the states for Medicaid differs from state to state based on each state's program. Federal funding averages 43 percent of program cost. Program costs over that level need to be funded within each state's operating budget.

The most widely known Medicaid coverage program is long-term-care coverage for the elderly who have exhausted their financial resources. Medicaid also provides coverage for a wide variety of healthcare programs for both the elderly and nonelderly. Coverage for medical services for nonelderly adults is based on each state's income guidelines for eligibility for public assistance. Federal guidelines require that children are eligible for coverage with family income up to 100 percent of the federal poverty level (133 percent for children of preschool age). Coverage for children was expanded in 1997 with the **Children's Health Insurance Program (CHIP)**. Under the CHIP program, most states have included children from families earning up to 200 percent of the poverty level.

CHIP is a joint partnership between the federal government and states, the District of Columbia (D.C.), and five U.S. territories to help provide children under age 19 from low- and moderate-income households with health insurance coverage and access to health care. In Fiscal Year (FY) 2020, the CMS Office of the Actuary estimated that 9.1 million individuals received health insurance funded through CHIP. As the largest single health payer in the United States, the CMS administers Medicare, Medicaid, CHIP, and the marketplaces. More than 148 million Americans rely on CMS programs for high-quality health coverage. The President's FY 2022 Budget estimates $1.4 trillion in mandatory and discretionary outlays for CMS, a net increase of $96 billion above FY 2021 enacted.

Figure 2-3 shows the total federal spending on Medicaid, CHIP, Medicare, and other health insurance programs.

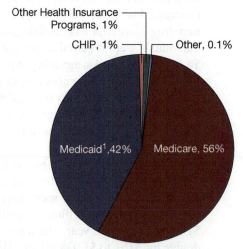

Other Health Insurance Programs, 1%

CHIP, 1% — Other, 0.1%

Medicaid[1],42%   Medicare, 56%

[1] Medicaid represents total Federal spending only

Figure 2-3 Federal Spending Dollars
Source: https://www.hhs.gov/about/budget/fy2022/index.html

Medicaid and CHIP cover an estimated 20 percent of the nonelderly population and serve as the largest insurer of children's health care after employer-sponsored health plans. Medicaid and CHIP expenditures totaled $345.7 billion in 2009, the latest year of available data. These costs will increase under the 2010 healthcare reform, with provisions of the new legislation increasing the income threshold for all beneficiaries to 138 percent of the poverty level in 2014.

Comprehension Check 2.2

In questions 1 to 3, identify if the healthcare insurance option is Medicaid, Medicare, or CHIP.

1. Ava Kelm just turned 65 years old. She is concerned about how she will be able to afford surgery on her leg. Her physician explained that she will have to stay overnight and have several medical tests run. Under which type of insurance will Ava be covered?

2. Luca Biel has had difficulty finding a full-time job. He has been working at the hospital as a part-time patient care assistant. He is making just enough to cover the bills with nothing left over. He cannot afford health insurance for his two children and is worried about it. What type of insurance may be an option for his children?

3. Jennifer Brown had a stroke recently and she can no longer care for herself. She has used all her financial resources to cover the assisted living expenses. What may be an insurance option for her to consider?

Healthcare Insurance for Members of the Armed Forces

TRICARE insurance provides healthcare insurance benefits for active members of the U.S. Armed Forces, retired military and National Guard and Reserve members, and their dependents. Until the mid-1950s, medical services for current and retired military and their families were provided at military healthcare facilities managed by the Veteran's Administration (VA). The medical needs of World War II and Korean War veterans and their families proved to be greater than the military services available, and Congress provided for the creation of a civilian counterpart to military healthcare services, creating the **Civilian Health and Medical Program of the Uniformed Services (CHAMPUS)** in 1966. CHAMPUS supplemented, rather than replaced, medical facilities run by the VA. The VA continues to be active in meeting the healthcare needs of members of the armed forces, both retired and active.

More than 9 million people are eligible to receive health care through TRICARE, a program run by the Department of Defense's (DoD) Military Health System. Among its beneficiaries are 1.5 million members of the active military and the other uniformed services (such as the Coast Guard), certain reservists, retired military personnel, and their qualified family members. The costs of that health care have been among the fastest-growing portions of the defense budget over the past 17 years, more than doubling in real (inflation-adjusted) terms since 2001. In 2017, DoD spent about $50 billion for health care. Much of the cost increases are attributable to new and expanded healthcare benefits and financial incentives to use those benefits.

TRICARE is the successor organization to CHAMPUS, providing healthcare insurance today to 9.2 million eligible beneficiaries through a series of programs:

- **TRICARE Standard** is a basic fee-for-service insurance program, allowing beneficiaries to use any civilian healthcare provider and requiring payments of deductibles and copayments.

- **TRICARE Extra** is a preferred provider arrangement, providing beneficiaries with lower out-of-pocket costs to use medical facilities enrolled in the program.

    • **TRICARE Prime** is an HMO model open to beneficiaries.

    • **TRICARE Reserve Select** and **TRICARE Reserve Retired** expanded the program to cover qualified active and retired members of the National Guard and Reserves.

Under the original TRICARE program, active and retired military were automatically dropped from eligibility when they qualified for Medicare coverage at age 65. Medicare benefits are not as comprehensive as TRICARE, and many veterans and their spouses found they needed to purchase a Medicare supplement plan with their own funds or face greater out-of-pocket costs. To address growing complaints in this area, Congress approved **TRICARE For Life** in 2001. This program takes those costs that would have been the responsibility of the patient under Medicare and transfers them to TRICARE for payment.

Knowledge Check

2.3

1. Individuals are eligible to receive Medicare benefits upon reaching age:
   A. 62 with limited benefits
   B. 65
   C. 66
   D. None of the above

2. Individuals are eligible to receive Medicaid benefits upon reaching age:
   A. 62 with limited benefits
   B. 65
   C. 66
   D. None of the above

3. Medicare Part C, providing for Medicare Advantage (MA) plans, was authorized by which of the following pieces of legislation?
   A. The Social Security Amendments of 1965
   B. The Balanced Budget Act of 1997
   C. The Medicare Prescription Drug, Improvement, and Modernization Act of 2003
   D. The Social Security Act of 1935

4. Medicare Part D was authorized by:
   A. The Social Security Amendments of 1965
   B. The Balanced Budget Act of 1997
   C. The Medicare Prescription Drug, Improvement, and Modernization Act of 2003
   D. The Social Security Act of 1935

5. TRICARE covers which of the following groups:
   A. Active and retired military
   B. Dependents of active and retired military
   C. Elected members of Congress
   D. Qualified National Guard and Reserve members
   E. All of the above
   F. All of the above *except* C

The Growing Uninsured

"The number of nonelderly uninsured Americans rose to 50.0 million in 2009—an increase of 4.3 million—amidst rising unemployment rates and an economic recession."

(The Kaiser Commission on Medicaid and the Uninsured, the Henry J. Kaiser Family Foundation, www.kff.org, December 2010)

A similar study by the U.S. Census Bureau shows the number of Americans without health insurance growing every year, from 38 million in 2000 to 46 million in 2008. The Census Bureau reports a total of 50.7 million uninsured in 2009 but confirms the cause of the increase resulting from the spike in unemployment in the recent recession. Workers have the right to exercise COBRA protections to continue work-based health insurance for up to 18 months following separation from employment but are required to pay the full cost of premiums. For many Americans left unemployed in the recession, their financial resources did not allow for paying healthcare premiums.

Compounding the impact of the unemployed on the number of people without health insurance is the growing number of the employed without insurance. Employers, faced with continuously rising premium costs, choose to drop health insurance as an employee benefit or employ more part-time employees who do not enjoy the same or any health insurance coverage as full-time employees. Employers attract and retain employees with a competitive pay and benefits package; in a tight employment market, they have the ability to reduce benefits without sacrificing the quality of their workforce. The latest available study on the uninsured was issued by the Kaiser Commission on Medicaid and the Uninsured in late 2010. More than one in five adults under age 65 was uninsured in 2009.

Uncompensated Care

There is an obvious direct correlation between the rise in the number of Americans without healthcare insurance and the volume of uncompensated care provided by the medical industry.

The Health and Human Services data show the number of uninsured has decreased from 2010 to 2016. In addition, the report also shows the number of nonelderly uninsured adults decreased by 41 percent, falling from 48.2 million to 28.2 million. All 50 states and the District of Columbia have experienced reductions in their uninsured rates since the implementation of the Affordable Care Act (ACA), with states that expanded Medicaid experiencing the largest reduction in their uninsured rate. California, Kentucky, New York, Oregon, Rhode Island, Washington, and West Virginia have reduced their uninsured rate by at least half from 2013 to 2019 through enrollment in marketplace coverage and expansion of Medicaid to adult populations.

The American Hospital Association estimates that for 2009, uncompensated care for hospitals reached $39 billion, or 6 percent of expenses. For the uninsured without the ability to pay privately for medical care, the hospital emergency room has become a substitute for the family physician, handling medical issues that would be addressed in a physician office for those with healthcare insurance.

The true costs of uncompensated care may be seen in more human terms. The uninsured:

- Receive less preventive care than those with insurance

- Delay medical attention to the point where the initial diagnosis is made at a more advanced stage of illness

- Are provided with less therapeutic care and have higher mortality rates after a diagnosis is made

Key Concepts

- Healthcare costs are growing and consuming more of our nation's resources.

- Managed care models such as preferred provider organizations and health maintenance organizations are the predominant model for health insurance.

- The enactment of COBRA in 1997 provided a way for employees to continue their health insurance when they change jobs or when they lose their job.

- Medicare, enacted in 1965, provides healthcare coverage for those citizens over the age of 65. Several amendments to the law have provided those covered with a wide variety of benefits.

- Medicaid, also enacted in 1965, provides healthcare coverage for the very poor and children. The Children's Health Insurance Program (CHIP) has provided an opportunity for many children to have basic health insurance.

- Both Medicare and Medicaid costs have been rising. Medicare will be affected by the large number of people eligible for Medicare beginning in 2011. Medicaid has been affected by the recession and high unemployment rate in the country.

- The U.S. military provides coverage for both its active and retired personnel.

- The increase in the uninsured population is contributing to the increase in uncompensated costs. Individuals without health insurance seek care in high-cost emergency rooms and sometimes only at a more advanced stage of illness.

The Rising Costs of Medical Services and Healthcare Reform

Key Terms

American Rescue Plan Act of 2021 (ARP)

Baby boomers

Build Back Better Plan

Clinton Health Care Plan of 1993

Massachusetts Health Care Reform Law of 2006

Oregon Health Plan

Patient Protection and Affordable Care Act of 2010 (PPACA)

Recovery Audit Contractor (RAC) Program

Severability clause

Tort

Tort reform

Chapter Objectives

After completing this chapter, readers should be able to:

- Identify and explain the major factors influencing the rising costs in health care.

- Discuss the history of universal health care in the United States, culminating in the Patient Protection and Affordable Care Act of 2010 (PPACA).

- Identify the major components of PPACA and the specifics of its implementation through 2022.

- Explain the financial coverage that the Build Back Better Act will provide

Chapter Glossary

American Rescue Plan Act of 2021 provides additional relief to address the continued impact of COVID-19 (i.e., coronavirus disease 2019) on the economy, public health, state and local governments, individuals, and businesses.

Baby boomers are members of the generation born between 1946 and 1964.

Build Back Better Act provides funding, establishes programs, and otherwise modifies provisions relating to a broad array of areas, including education, labor, child care, health care, taxes, immigration, and the environment.

The **Clinton Health Care Plan of 1993** was the failed attempt to secure universal healthcare coverage for all Americans.

The **Massachusetts Health Care Reform Law of 2006** was state legislation providing universal healthcare coverage for all citizens of the state of Massachusetts.

The **Oregon Health Plan** was the first attempt by a state government to implement universal health care.

The **Patient Protection and Affordable Care Act of 2010 (PPACA)** is landmark healthcare reform, requiring most Americans to purchase healthcare insurance and expanding coverage requirements of existing group health insurance plans.

The **Recovery Audit Contractor (RAC) Program** is as public-private partnership designed to uncover improper payments in the Medicare and Medicaid programs.

A **severability clause** is included in legislation and states that if any one section of the law is later ruled illegal, the balance of the law remains in full force and effect.

A **tort** is a civil legal action arising from a wrongful act that results in the injury to someone's person, reputation, or property.

Tort reform is the process to contain medical malpractice costs and is designed to place limits on noneconomic and punitive damages, limit attorney fees, and shorten the statute of limitations for filing legal claims.

The Rising Costs of Medical Services

Health care is expensive and continues to become more expensive. Annual increases in the cost of health care exceed the increases in the cost-of-living index. Even with inflation lower than average as a result of the current recession, the U.S. Bureau of Labor Statistics reports that cost increases for medical services rose 3.4 percent in the 12 months ending November 30, 2010, compared to the cost-of-living increase for all items of just 1.1 percent. Since 1960, increases in healthcare spending have consumed an ever greater share of the country's gross domestic product as evidenced in Figure 3-1.

In this report, personal healthcare expenditures rose from $23.3 billion in 1960 to over $2 trillion in 2009. Expenditures represent personal healthcare costs, regardless of the source of payment for services. Healthcare spending is expected to rise 6.5 percent in 2022 as the industry tries to stable out after the choppy seas of the COVID-19 pandemic.

The choices consumers make affect the level of services provided and costs. Patients may become claustrophobic in a closed MRI and demand the use of the open MRI, which is newer technology and purchased by the facility at a cost exceeding $500,000. The facility's competitor across town is faced with the dilemma of either investing an equal amount in the new technology or losing business. A pharmaceutical company brings a new drug to market and invests heavily in advertising in the public media, encouraging patients to contact their physicians for a prescription. Chronic conditions that previously would have led to an early death are now treatable and extend life but at the cost of increased demands on the medical system.

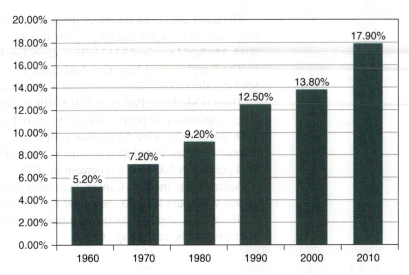

Figure 3-1 Personal Healthcare Expenditures as Percentage of GDP
Source: Data from Centers for Medicare & Medicaid Services; www.cms.gov/NationalHealthExpend-Data/25_NHE_Fact_Sheet.asp

Additional cost pressures in the medical industry come from the need to recruit and retain highly trained professionals at a time when there continues to be shortages in a number of specialties. Fraud and abuse in the system add to medical costs, as do the involvement of the legal process in medical malpractice. The following sections will explore these issues in more detail.

Baby Boomers and Life Expectancy

January 1, 2011, marked a major milestone in healthcare financing: the first of the **baby boomers** turned 65 and became eligible for Medicare. Baby boomers, those born between 1946 and 1964, have been a major force in society since they were born. Schools were overcrowded in the 1950s, antiwar and antiestablishment protests marked the 1960s, and the "boomers" dominated the labor force in the 1980s and 1990s, limiting opportunities for promotion for members of Generations X and Y. In 2008, the first of the baby boomers turned 62 and were eligible for Social Security.

Social Security was approved in 1935, promising retirement income to individuals over age 65. Full Social Security benefits are available to individuals who have contributed to the system for a minimum of 40 calendar quarters (10 years). Individuals meeting the 40-quarter eligibility rule are also allowed early retirement at age 62 with reduced benefits.

A biological male born in 1930 had a life expectancy of 58 years; a biological female, 62 years. Given those life expectancies, Social Security was not seen to be a major expense for the federal government and easily financed by payroll taxes established as part of the program. In 1965, the year Medicare was approved, life expectancy had increased to 70.2 years. In 2008, the World Bank Development Indicators placed U.S. life expectancy at 78.4 years. The normal life-cycle process demands more from the medical system as an individual ages. With more elderly Americans, the need for medical services and related costs will continue to rise.

The U.S. Census Bureau numbered the members of the baby boomer generation at 78 million in 2009, fully 25 percent of the total U.S. population of 307 million. This vast number of individuals becoming eligible for Medicare between 2011 and 2029, compounded by their longer life expectancy, will place enormous pressure on the government's ability to meet the financing needs of programs for older adults.

N
and
201
T
SNA
T
anc
I
Bur
12.4
A
cen
S
boo

In

T
A
of d
mer
incr
Dru
a de
I
for
pul
F
forr
app
thro
T
tecl
ness
the
to r
T
inc

In October 2018, a doctor in Kentucky was found guilty of healthcare fraud and sentenced to three years and six months in prison and ordered to pay $257,515 in restitution. The doctor defrauded Medicare, Medicaid, and other insurers by implanting medically unnecessary pacemakers in patients, causing unnecessary procedures and follow-up care to be billed to health insurance programs. Between 2007 and 2011, the doctor implanted approximately 234 pacemakers in patients at St. Joseph London hospital. Dozens of those patients' pacemakers were medically unnecessary under well-established national guidelines and Medicare coverage rules.

In November 2018, a pharmacist and marketer was sentenced to 16 months in prison after pleading guilty for his involvement in a compounding prescription scheme to defraud government healthcare benefit programs, including TRICARE. To date, 11 people have been charged and 8 convicted for the largest healthcare fraud scheme ever investigated and prosecuted in Mississippi.

In April 2019, a former medical doctor and his business partner were each sentenced to 33 months in prison in Nevada for their roles in a $7.1 million Medicare healthcare fraud scheme that occurred at three Las Vegas hospice and home healthcare agencies. The defendants filed false enrollment documents with Medicare to enable the former doctor to operate hospice and home care agencies through nominees despite his prior exclusion from all federal healthcare programs. Furthermore, they submitted fraudulent hospice care claims for people who were not terminally ill and did not require hospice care.

Estimates on the annual losses to Medicare and Medicaid from fraud and abuse vary widely. There is, however, a consensus that improper payments result in billions of dollars lost annually by these programs. To combat these problems, the Centers for Medicare and Medicaid Services (CMS) have enlisted the services of the private sector in the **Recovery Audit Contractor (RAC) Program**. Independent contractors work for CMS and are reimbursed with a percentage of program overpayments that are recovered by the audits. The RAC Program was first initiated as a trial program in the **Medicare Modernization Act** of 2003 and made permanent in the **Tax Relief and Healthcare Act of 2006.** The mission of the RAC Program is to:

- Conduct provider audits to detect and correct billing errors

- Train providers in proper methods of claim submission to avoid future errors

- Lower the error rate in CMS programs

- Protect taxpayers and future program beneficiaries by ensuring that only appropriate costs are reimbursed

Claims for reimbursement under the CMS programs are deemed to be improper for a number of reasons. The most common reasons for disallowed claims come from claims that are improperly coded, claims for services that are considered to be medically unnecessary, or claims with insufficient documentation. Program providers with disallowed claims have four options for reimbursing the program: payment by check for the improperly received payments, allowing CMS to recover the amounts due from future program payments, negotiating a payment plan with the CMS, or appealing the disallowed claims. From the beginning of the program in 2006 through March 2008, over $900 million in overpayments have been collected through these audits.

In Fiscal Year (FY) 2016, Medicare Fee-For-Service (FFS) RACs collectively identified and corrected 380,229 claims with improper payments that resulted in $473.92 million in improper payments being corrected. The total corrections identified included $404.46 million in overpayments collected and $69.46 million in underpayments repaid to providers. This represents a 7.5 percent increase from program corrections in FY 2015, which were $440.69 million. Table 3-1 shows the total amount of collections from the RACs.

Table 3-1 Total Collected Payments

	CORRECTIONS BY RAC					
	Overpayments Collected		Underpayments Restored		Total Corrected	
RAC	**No. of Claims**	**Amount Collected**	**No. of Claims**	**Amount Restored**	**No. of Claims**	**Amount Corrected**
Performant	72,681	$56,259,974.80	6,258	$9,582,298.15	78,939	$65,842,272.95
CGI	63,866	$44,544,053.62	1,096	$3,402,728.33	64,962	$47,946,781.95
Cotiviti	69,385	$143,213,553.28	25,781	$38,461,475.66	95,166	$181,675,028.94
HDI	134,099	$160,389,190.28	6,492	$18,007,417.08	140,591	$178,396,607.36
Unknown[15]	565	$56,657.91	6	$5,606.16	571	$62,264.07
Total	*340,596*	*$404,463,429.89*	*39,633*	*$69,459,525.38*	*380,229*	*$473,922,955.27*

[15] Due to changing MAC workload numbers, these claims could not be attributed to a specific RAC in the Data Warehouse. No RAC has been paid contingency fees for the correction of these claims.
Source: Recovery Auditing in Medicare Fee For-Service for Fiscal Year 2016.

The Costs of Medical Malpractice

Medical professionals, like anyone else, can make mistakes. However, mistakes in the medical field can cause serious injury or death. In many instances, such mistakes result in a lawsuit, with either a settlement or a jury verdict awarding cash damages to the injured party. Medical professionals—not just physicians but others such as nurses and pharmacists—purchase medical malpractice insurance to protect themselves and their businesses from the financial impact of a medical mistake.

BOX 3-1 Legal Cases in Medical Malpractice

A woman in Indiana underwent heart bypass surgery and a surgical pad was overlooked in the incision, adhering to her heart. A second surgery was performed, and the woman died from perforations to the heart leading to multiple-organ failure. The jury awarded $2.2 million for wrongful death.

A New York woman gave birth to a girl in 1984. The baby suffered brain damage from oxygen deprivation that caused cerebral palsy, confining the girl to a wheelchair for the rest of her life. A jury in 2009 awarded the amount of $43.5 million.

In 2009, a New York woman received a jury award in the amount of $60 million when she sued for disfigurement and other damages resulting from a procedure to remove excess skin from her thigh following her successful loss of a large amount of weight. Expert medical witnesses were able to convince the jury that she suffered vaginal deformation and other medical conditions that she would have for life.

In the private sector, many employees and their families are covered by group health insurance plans from employers. People not covered by employer-sponsored plans or eligible for government programs either purchase individual policies or are uninsured.

Chapter 2 included a discussion of the political realities that resulted in major changes to the financing of entitlements. President Roosevelt's New Deal brought income to older Americans through Social Security. President Johnson's Great Society brought health-care protection to older and low-income Americans through Medicare and Medicaid. The next great debate on health care has centered on universal healthcare coverage.

The Oregon Health Plan

In 1989, the state of Oregon became the first state to move toward universal health-care coverage with the **Oregon Health Plan**. The plan had two major components: a requirement that employers provide healthcare insurance for their employees and the expansion of the state's Medicaid program to cover all residents below the poverty line. The employer mandate never received a required federal waiver and was not imple-mented. The Medicaid expansion also required a federal waiver, signed by President Bill Clinton in March 1993. The Oregon Health Plan included a unique rationing plan for medical services to contain the costs of expanding the number of individuals covered by the program.

Under the Oregon rationing plan, a list of common medical conditions and related treatments was prepared. Treatments were prioritized based on the costs of treatments and effectiveness in improving patient health and life expectancies. In the state's two-year budgeting process, Oregon would budget funds for the program and determine a cutoff point on the list. Treatments above the cutoff point would be approved for plan reimbursement of medical costs, and treatments below the cutoff point would be denied coverage.

The Oregon Health Plan enrolled almost 120,000 in 1994, the first year of operation of the program. The plan continues to be in place, with increasing treatment costs and budget constraints limiting both treatments covered by the plan and plan enrollment.

The Clinton Health Care Plan of 1993

"Millions of Americans are just a pink slip away from losing their health insur-ance, and one serious illness away from losing all their savings. Millions more are locked into the jobs they now have just because they or someone in their families has once been sick and they have what is called the preexisting condi-tion. And on any given day, over 37 million Americans—most of them working people and their little children—have no health insurance at all. And in spite of all this, our medical bills are growing at over twice the rate of inflation, and the United States spends over a third more of its income on health care than any other nation on earth."

(President Bill Clinton, addressing a joint session of Congress, September 22, 1993. http://millercenter.org/president/speeches/detail/3926)

In the months prior to November 1992, Bill Clinton was running for president as the nominee of the Democratic Party, with healthcare reform a key platform issue. After his successful election, President Clinton moved quickly, establishing the Task Force on National Health Care Reform. The task force was led by then–First Lady Hillary Rodham Clinton (later elected a U.S. senator and then appointed as secretary of state in the Obama administration).

The **Clinton Health Care Plan of 1993**, dubbed "HillaryCare" by opponents, which was picked up by the media, would have required all American citizens and permanent resident aliens to be a member of a healthcare program. Employers would have been required to offer healthcare coverage to employees, and regional healthcare alliances would have been established to provide healthcare insurance to the currently uninsured. Physicians and healthcare facilities were to be reimbursed on an FFS basis. Premiums for insurance coverage would be subsidized by the federal government for those with low incomes, and maximum annual out-of-pocket costs would be established. The program would have been administered by the states, with funding provided by the federal government.

The Clinton Plan failed due to attack by Republicans as an unneeded intrusion of the government into health care and by a lack of Democratic unity in support of the program. By the summer of 1994, Congress recognized that the program had no chance of passage even in a compromised form and abandoned it.

Massachusetts Health Care Reform Law of 2006

The state of Massachusetts moved forward with universal health care for residents of that state with the approval of the **Massachusetts Health Care Reform Law of 2006**, known as MassHealth. Effective in 2007, employers with 11 or more employees were required to provide healthcare insurance programs for their employees or pay a fine of up to $295 per employee. Individuals without access to employer group insurance plans were required to purchase insurance through one of seven state-approved programs in the Commonwealth Care Health Connector or pay a fine of approximately $1,000 annually.

Similar to the federal program of 2010, the MassHealth plan provides for premiums on a sliding scale based on family income. Families earning less than 150 percent of the federal poverty level receive healthcare benefits without premiums, and subsidized premiums are available to families of four earning up to approximately $66,000 a year. Medicaid coverage for children has been expanded to cover children in families earning up to 300 percent of the federal poverty level.

MassHealth provided healthcare insurance to a great majority of the state's residents in 2010. In the year 2022, MassHealth is still in existence. MassHealth provides coverage to approximately two million people.

The Patient Protection and Affordable Care Act of 2010 (PPACA)

On February 26, 2009, President Obama delivered his budget message to Congress, outlining a set of eight principles for transforming and modernizing America's healthcare system. He stated that he expected that his office and Congress would work together over the coming year to pass meaningful healthcare reform legislation. His eight principles for healthcare reform were itemized as:

1. **Protect families' financial health.** Americans and American businesses must be protected from annual increases in the cost of healthcare insurance.

2. **Make health coverage affordable.** Inefficiencies must be eliminated from the healthcare system, such as excessive administrative costs and unnecessary tests.

3. **Universality.** Healthcare reform needs to set a plan that will result in all Americans having healthcare coverage.

4. **Portability of coverage.** The plan needs to include provisions that will guarantee continued coverage when an individual changes employment, while being ensured that preexisting conditions will be covered.

5. **Choice guarantees.** Reform needs to include the opportunity for individuals to have a choice of health insurance plans and physicians. Employer-based health-care insurance plans should remain in place and be available to employees.

6. **Invest in wellness and prevention.** The plan must include funding for proven programs to address societal healthcare issues such as smoking, obesity, and a sedentary lifestyle.

7. **Patient safety and quality care.** Incentives need to be provided in the plan to implement procedures for patient safety that have been proven to be successful. The plan must also provide for improvements in health information technology.

8. **Fiscal sustainability.** Lowering the annual cost increases in health care, productivity improvements, and revenues from sources such as premiums from currently uninsured Americans must provide for the plan to pay for itself.

President Obama made effective use of Democratic majorities in both the Senate and House of Representatives to push through healthcare reform with the passage of the **Patient Protection and Affordable Care Act of 2010 (PPACA)**. This caused a major shift in affordability for health insurance and is impactful in future trends in meeting an individual's health care needs.

The first part of the comprehensive health care reform law was enacted on March 23, 2010. The law was amended by the Health Care and Education Reconciliation Act on March 30, 2010. The name "Affordable Care Act (ACA)" is usually used to refer to the final, amended version of the law. (It's sometimes known as "PPACA," "ACA," or "Obamacare.")

The law provides numerous rights and protections that make health coverage more fair and easy to understand, along with subsidies (through "premium tax credits" and "cost-sharing reductions") to make it more affordable.

The law also expands the Medicaid program to cover more people with low incomes.

This new law, popularly known as "ObamaCare," was designed to bring affordable healthcare protection to many, but not all, of the millions of Americans currently without healthcare insurance, as well as improving health insurance coverage for individuals currently covered under group health plans. The ranks of the uninsured have grown from the estimated 37 million at the time President Clinton addressed the joint session of Congress on health care in 1993 to over 50 million in 2010.

Provisions of PPACA: 2010

"March 23, 2010 after almost a century of trying; after over a year of debate; health insurance reforms became law in the United States of America."

(www.whitehouse.gov/the-press-office/remarks-president-and-vice-president-signing-health-insurance-reform-bill)

Documentation provided to Congress as part of the PPACA legislation came in at a total of 2,841 pages. The final law fundamentally reshaped health insurance coverage for Americans and contained literally hundreds of individual provisions. Students desiring more detailed information on the act than is provided in this overview are referred to an excellent summary prepared by the Henry J. Kaiser Family Foundation at *https://www.kff.org/health-reform/*.

Most of the changes under PPACA were implemented in 2014, but a number of provisions were effective on October 1, 2010:

• A temporary high-risk insurance pool was created to provide health insurance coverage for individuals with preexisting conditions who have been without insurance for a period of at least 6 months.

• Coverage for dependent children under all individual and group insurance contracts was expanded to cover dependent children until age 26. While a number of states already had this provision, this rule now applies nationwide.

- The lifetime maximum for cost reimbursement was eliminated. Many policies had a lifetime cap on coverage for the treatment of costly diseases such as cancer of $1 million or even less. The legislation does allow for some grandfathering of limits that were in place prior to March 23, 2010.

- Annual limits on cost reimbursement were also eliminated. For 2010, annual limits were restricted, with full prohibition of annual limits effective in 2014.

- Children cannot be excluded from coverage under their parents' account for preexisting conditions. The only requirement is that children will need to be added during open enrollment periods.

- Medical services categorized as preventive care, such as immunizations, mammograms, and colonoscopies were required to be paid by the insurance company in full.

- Healthcare insurance providers were prohibited from canceling insurance coverage, except in the case of fraud.

- Individuals covered by Medicare and meeting certain conditions receive a one-time $250 payment to assist in paying for the cost of prescriptions not covered under Medicare Part D.

- A 10 percent tax was levied on the services of indoor tanning salons.

Provisions of PPACA: 2011

- Annual fees imposed on manufacturers of pharmaceuticals.

- Changes were made to tax-free medical spending accounts.

- Funding is now provided for community health centers to address the medical needs of low-income individuals.

- The act addressed the "doughnut hole" in Medicare Part D coverage for prescriptions, where currently recipients are required to pay for a portion of the costs of their medications.

- $50 million was provided to states to develop programs for tort reform.

Provisions of PPACA: 2012 and 2013

- New annual fees were imposed on the pharmaceutical industry.

- A $2,500 annual limit was placed on flexible spending accounts.

- The requirement on itemized deductions for personal income taxes that medical expenses exceed 7.5 percent of adjusted gross income was amended to allow deductions of medical expenses only in excess of 10 percent of adjusted gross income.

- Individuals earning over $200,000 and married couples earning over $250,000 saw an increase in the Medicare tax from the current 1.45 percent to 2.35 percent; the amount of unearned income on tax returns with these higher levels was subject to a Medicare tax of 3.8 percent.

Provisions of PPACA: 2014

The full impact of health insurance reform was implemented in 2014:

- Healthcare exchanges were created to be run by individual states to provide healthcare insurance for the uninsured.

- All Americans were required to have healthcare insurance or pay a fine. Federal subsidies assisted in the purchase of healthcare insurance for people with lower incomes.

- Companies with 50 or more employees were provided group healthcare insurance for its employees or pay fines for noncompliance.

- Medicaid coverage was expanded for low-income individuals under age 65.

- Revenue for the program was generated by new fees on health insurance companies.

Provisions of PPACA: 2015–2018

Final implementation of the program was scheduled for 2015–2018:

- Annual increases in fees for pharmaceutical and healthcare insurance companies and increased penalties on the uninsured are now in place.

- In 2018, there was a new 40 percent *excise tax* on the most expensive group healthcare programs ("Cadillac plans"). An excise tax is a tax imposed on any specific product, in this case group healthcare programs. Excise taxes are also used to tax items such as gasoline and tobacco products.

The law provided numerous rights and protections that make health coverage more fair and easy to understand, along with subsidies (through "premium tax credits" and "cost-sharing reductions") to make it more affordable.

The law expanded the Medicaid program to cover more people with low incomes.

Provisions of PPACA: 2019–2022

PPACA is still implemented today and is known as the Affordable Care Act. There were a record number of people signed up under the Affordable Care Act by November 1, 2021:

- 14 million people signed up for health insurance under the Affordable Care Act.

- More subsidies are available making insurance premiums lower.

- However, due to changes within the political sector, financial assistance may disappear at the end of 2022 if Congress doesn't renew the policies approved in the 2021 COVID-19 relief package.

The future of health care resides in the decision made during the congressional discussions.

The additional subsidies will expire on December. 31, 2022, unless Congress approves President Biden's **Build Back Better Plan**, which would extend these subsidies through 2025.

The Build Back Better Plan will impact health care in several ways:

- The framework will reduce premiums for more than 9 million Americans who buy insurance through the Affordable Care Act Marketplace by an average of $600 per person per year. For example, a family of four earning $80,000 per year would save nearly $3,000 per year (or $246 per month) on health insurance premiums. Experts predict that more than 3 million people who would otherwise be uninsured will gain health insurance.

- The Build Back Better Plan will deliver health care coverage through Affordable Care Act premium tax credits to up to 4 million uninsured people in states that have been denied Medicaid coverage. A 40-year old in the coverage gap would have to pay $450 per month for benchmark coverage—more than half of their income in many cases. The framework provides individuals $0 premiums, finally making health care affordable and accessible.

- The Build Back Better framework will expand Medicare coverage to cover hearing coverage, so that older Americans can access the affordable care they need. *https://www.whitehouse.gov/build-back-better/*

The American Rescue Plan (ARP) enhanced and expanded marketplace premium tax credits under the Affordable Care Act.

- President Biden signed the **American Rescue Plan Act of 2021 (ARP)** into law on March 11, 2021. ARP makes major improvements in access to and affordability of health coverage through the marketplace by increasing eligibility for financial assistance to help pay for marketplace coverage.

- The new law lowered premiums for most people who currently have a marketplace health plan and expands access to financial assistance for more consumers.

- Under the new law, many people who bought their own health insurance directly through the marketplace became eligible to receive increased tax credits to reduce their premiums. Beginning on April 1, 2021, consumers enrolling in marketplace coverage through HealthCare.gov were able to take advantage of these increased savings and lower costs.

- Premiums after these new savings decreased, on average, by $50 per person per month or by $85 per policy per month. Four out of five enrollees are now able to find a plan for $10 or less/month after premium tax credits, and over 50 percent can now find a Silver plan for $10 or less.

The benefits of the ARP are:

- About 14.9 million Americans who currently lack health insurance can save money on their premiums to find the coverage they need at a price they can afford.

- 3.6 million uninsured people are now eligible for healthcare coverage savings.

- 1.8 million uninsured people are now eligible for zero-dollar benchmark.

- An additional 9.5 million uninsured people with incomes between 150 percent and 400 percent of the federal poverty level (FPL) now qualify for additional financial support to reduce out-of-pocket costs for marketplace premiums.

The COVID-19 pandemic has exacerbated stark health disparities among certain racial and ethnic minority populations in several areas, including infections, hospitalizations, death rates, and vaccination rates. Many of these same populations have experienced job loss or loss of health insurance coverage at disproportionately high rates.

- 48,000 uninsured American Indians and Alaska Natives are now eligible to save money on healthcare coverage, and 21,000 are eligible for zero-dollar benchmark marketplace plans.

- 730,000 uninsured Latinos are eligible to save money on healthcare coverage, and 580,000 will be eligible for zero-dollar benchmark marketplace plans.

- 360,000 uninsured black and African Americans are eligible to save money on healthcare coverage, and 328,000 will be eligible for zero-dollar benchmark marketplace plans.

- 197,000 uninsured Asians, Native Hawaiians, and Pacific Islanders are eligible to save money on healthcare coverage, and 50,000 will be eligible for zero-dollar benchmark marketplace plans.

Comprehension Check 3.1

1. Ashley Jones was in college studying to become a medical assistant, while working at her local bakery. She was fortunate that she was 1 of 120,000 in 1994 to be insured for universal healthcare coverage based on the cost of her treatment and medical services. Which state was she living in during 1994?

2. A dentist in Massachusetts had 15 employees including dental assistants, dental hygienists, and front office staff. Because the dentist did not provide healthcare insurance for their employees, what could their maximum fine be based on having 15 employees and not providing their employees with insurance programs?

3. Mr. Duwl's son has a condition that he was born with that impacts his breathing. He is concerned under the Patient Protection and Affordable Act provision that his son will not be covered. What provision will his son be covered under?

4. Tom Savy is trying to explain the benefits of the American Rescue Plan to a friend. What are three benefits of the plan that Tom could explain as benefits of the plan?

Accountable Care Organizations

One of the keys to cost containment that assists in paying for the program is lowering medical costs through the use of accountable care organizations (ACOs), a system for the delivery of medical services created by PPACA. Under this program, local hospitals form legal alliances with physicians and other healthcare professionals to coordinate patient care. Members of each ACO are held accountable for providing quality medical care and eliminating waste from the system. Waste in the context of health care is defined as system inefficiencies where care provided is redundant, ineffective, or contrary to medical best practices. ACOs generating positive results share in the savings from more effective care provided at lower costs.

All members of each ACO need to share patient information for the development of the most effective plan of care. Patients also have a role to play in cost containment: individual patients are involved in prevention and wellness programs, and each patient is assigned to a midlevel professional, such as a physician assistant (PA) or registered nurse (RN), as their first point of contact. These midlevel professionals operate in a similar fashion to gatekeepers in managed care, operating under the direction of the physician to provide medical services that do not need the direct involvement of the physician and handling over the phone any minor medical issues that do not require an office visit. Under MassHealth, Massachusetts General Hospital has had a functioning ACO since that state's healthcare program was adopted in 2006.

Political Opposition to Healthcare Reform

Just as President Obama was able to hold together his Democratic Party majority to ensure passage of PPACA, the Republicans were united in opposition. Disagreement between the two parties on the legislation was centered on the fiscal responsibility of the program. Financing the program calls for $500 billion in cost savings in Medicare expenditures over the next decade. Opponents have stated that that level of savings is not realistic, citing as evidence the track record of Congress in projecting Medicare costs. In 1965, upon the passage of the Medicare law, Congress projected that Medicare costs would reach $8 billion in 1990. Actual Medicare costs in 1990 were $67 billion.

In the 2022 midterm elections, the Republican party gains control of the House of Representatives. The democratic party gains control over the senate. Healthcare policy in 2023 will be influenced by the 2024 presidential election cycle, which began the moment the midterm elections ended. By the time Congress returns to start the 118th Congress, presidential politics will already be in play. https://www.natlawreview.com/article/way-too-early-preview-what-midterm-election-results-might-mean-health-policy-2023

Legal Opposition to Healthcare Reform

Political opposition to healthcare reform has also included an attack on the legislation on legal grounds.

Since 2010, various states, private entities, and individuals have challenged parts or all of the ACA nearly 2,000 times in state and federal courts. The following are brief summaries of court cases opposing the ACA.

Eighteen states—along with two individuals—filed a lawsuit in February 2018 arguing that, because federal lawmakers reduced the mandate's "shared responsibility payment" to $0 through the 2017 Tax Cuts and Jobs Act, the individual mandate is unconstitutional. This argument was based on the Supreme Court's 2012 ruling that the individual mandate was a tax. If the shared responsibility payment is $0, the individual mandate generates no money and, therefore, cannot be a tax, the challengers argued. The challengers also argued the rest of the health law cannot be "severed" from the individual mandate and, therefore, the entire ACA is unconstitutional.

Twenty-one states, along with the House of Representatives, defended the federal law, arguing that the individual mandate is constitutional—and that it is severable from the rest of the ACA if the Supreme Court were to rule that the mandate is unconstitutional. These states also challenged whether the states and individuals filing the lawsuit had standing to challenge the health law.

The federal government under the Trump Administration initially did not defend the ACA before the Supreme Court. The Department of Justice (DOJ) filed an amicus brief arguing the individual mandate is unconstitutional and the rest of the ACA cannot be severed and, therefore, is unconstitutional. Under the Biden Administration, the DOJ switched its position, arguing that the individual mandate is constitutional and severable from the rest of the health law.

The Supreme Court ruled in June 2021 that both the individual and state plaintiffs lacked standing to challenge the law in court because the plaintiffs failed to show a personal injury that was "fairly traceable" to the $0 individual mandate. Since the Court rejected the case based on standing, it did not discuss arguments relating to the constitutionality of the individual mandate and whether it is severable from the rest of the health law.

The federal government counters that the concept of mandatory insurance falls under the government's ability to regulate interstate commerce through the Commerce Clause. The Commerce Clause is found in Article 1, Section 8, Clause 3 of the U.S. Constitution. It states that Congress has the right "to regulate commerce with foreign nations, and among the several States, and with the Indian Tribes." The term *commerce* here refers to the conduct of business. Proponents of PPACA argue that the Commerce Clause provides the legal basis for the act.

More than 30 lawsuits have been filed seeking to overturn PPACA. Through the fall of 2010 and the winter of 2011, U.S. district courts across the country heard these cases. The final scorecard at the district court level was three courts upholding the act and two declaring it unconstitutional.

The U.S. legal process calls for appeals from district court decisions to be heard by one of the U.S. circuit courts of appeals. In June 2011, the Sixth Circuit Court of Appeals in Cincinnati, Ohio, ruled that the requirement for most Americans to have health insurance or pay a penalty is constitutional.

Two months later, the 11th Circuit Court of Appeals in Atlanta, Georgia, reached the opposite decision, ruling that mandatory health insurance is unconstitutional. An interesting legal point in the PPACA is that the legislation was drafted and approved without a **severability clause**. A severability clause states that if any one section of the law is later ruled illegal, the balance of the law remains in full force and effect and is commonly added to complex legislation. The Atlanta appeals court ruling also made the determination that the remainder of the Affordable Care Act, excluding the mandatory health insurance provision, could remain in force.

In September 2011, the 4th Circuit Court of Appeals in Richmond, Virginia, dismissed two challenges to the act on technical issues.

In one of the underlying cases, the 4th Circuit held that noncompliance fines imposed under the PPACA were taxes, not penalties. This interpretation is consistent with that of the Obama administration, and supports the conclusion that the individual mandate (and penalties for failing to comply with it) fall within Congress's authority under the Taxing and Spending clause of the Constitution.

Tax penalties were reduced to $0 at the end of 2018. In most states, people who have been uninsured since 2019 are no longer assessed a penalty.

But there are some areas of the country where penalties still apply if a person is uninsured and not eligible for an exemption.

As of 2022, there are penalties for being uninsured in Massachusetts, New Jersey, California, Rhode Island, and the District of Columbia.

Key Concepts

- Americans are living longer with chronic conditions that contribute to the continued increases in the cost of health care.

- New technology is expensive and may extend life for only a few weeks or months.

- The workforce in health care is one of the most highly educated of any industry. Additionally, training costs for qualified personnel adds to the general cost of health care.

- Fraud and abuse in healthcare reimbursement has been a problem for some time. Both the federal government and insurance companies are taking steps to reduce both. The RAC process is an example of how overpayments may be recovered due to error or fraud.

- Medical malpractice premiums continue to be of concern to providers.

- Over the last 15 years, many efforts to reform the healthcare system have been attempted. The Patient Protection and Affordable Care Act of 2010 is the latest attempt to reform the system.

Accounting For Healthcare Facilities

Accounting has been described as the language of business. Section II provides the reader with the basics of double-entry accounting and key accounting concepts. Individual accounting transactions are the building blocks that lead to the two primary accounting reports: the balance sheet and the income statement.

Basic Accounting Concepts

Key Terms

Accounting
Accounting equation
Accounts payable
Accounts receivable
Assets
Capital assets
Capital expenses
Credits
Debits
Double-entry accounting
Expenses
General ledger
Liabilities
Net worth
Operating expenses
Practice management systems (PMS)
Revenues
Trial balance

Chapter Objectives

After completing this chapter, readers should be able to:

- Define the terminology used in the language of accounting.

- Explain the basics of double-entry accounting, with every entry into the financial records requiring an equal and offsetting debit and credit.

- Describe the major differences between manual and computerized accounting systems.

Chapter Glossary

Accounting is a process, and the end product from this process is financial information.

An **accounting equation** is the equation used regularly in the accounting field in double-entry accounting. The equation can be written in several different ways, such as Assets = Liabilities + Net worth or Net worth = Assets − Liabilities.

Accounts payable is the amount owed by the medical facility for goods and services purchased on credit.

Accounts receivable is the cumulative balance of all of the individual charges for medical services due from patients and insurance companies not paid in cash at time of service.

Assets are the items of financial value owned by the medical facility.

Capital assets are items of higher than minimal value owned by the business, such as buildings and equipment, which have a relatively long, useful life.

Capital expenses are the annual costs related to the decline in value over time of assets with a relatively long, useful life.

Credits in double-entry accounting are used to post increases in revenue, liability, and equity accounts and to post decreases in asset and expense accounts.

Debits in double-entry accounting are used to post increases in asset and expense accounts and to post decreases in revenue, liability, and equity accounts.

Double-entry accounting requires that every individual entry into the financial system include one or more debits balanced and offset by one or more credits.

Expenses serve as a measurement of the resources used, such as personnel and supplies, to generate revenues.

A **general ledger** is the journal of original entry records for each day of events. This is shown as the date the transaction occurred.

Liabilities are what are owed by the medical facility for unpaid bills for goods and services and longer-term debt, such as balances on bank and equipment loans.

Net worth is the difference between total assets and total liabilities. Depending on the legal structure, terms used for net worth include owner's equity, capital stock and retained earnings, net assets, and fund balance.

Operating expenses are the costs involved in running the business on a daily basis.

Practice management systems (PMS) are comprehensive computer software programs designed specifically for medical offices.

Revenues are the amounts earned by the medical facility in providing services to patients and clients.

A **trial balance** is a listing of the current balances of all accounts in the financial system at a certain point in time to ensure that the total of the accounts with a debit balance equals the total of the accounts with a credit balance.

Introduction

A Franciscan friar, Luca Pacioli, first codified double-entry accounting in 1494, which continues to this day to serve as the foundation for modern accounting systems. Based on his articulation of the double-entry method of bookkeeping in his Summa, Pacioli is sometimes described as "the father of accounting." The Summa, which was published in 1494, is generally considered to contain the first printed (as opposed to handwritten) description of double-entry bookkeeping.

Accounting has been referred to as the language of business. Just as medicine has its own language, one that is foreign to people outside of the profession, the same is true of accounting. This chapter and the following two chapters on the balance sheet and the income statement are designed to provide the reader with a basic understanding of the language of accounting, the inputs and outputs of the accounting process, and the ability to read and understand financial statements of healthcare facilities. This brief overview will not turn the reader into a hospital chief financial officer, but it will provide some insights that the healthcare professional can benefit from in their work environment.

People outside of the world of financial management will commonly use the terms **bookkeeper** and **accountant** interchangeably. Bookkeeping tasks involve the recording of transactions into the financial records of the medical facility. Specific tasks that would fall under the heading of bookkeeping will include the cashier entering data on payments received from patients and the accounts payable clerk preparing vendor invoices for payment. The job responsibilities of an accountant are much broader and include reviewing and approving bookkeeping entries, preparing financial statements, presenting financial reports and analyses to top management, and designing and enforcing internal control procedures to safeguard the financial resources of the organization.

In the days of manual accounting systems, businesses would maintain a series of accounting records, called ledgers or journals, to record financial transactions. Modern computer technology has developed financial management software that has replaced the handwritten accounting records. These software programs have eliminated much of the repetitive manual work of maintaining the financial records of the medical facility. However, it continues to be the responsibility of bookkeeping and accounting staffs to ensure the accuracy of the records. The use of computerized accounting systems is discussed later in this chapter.

Double-Entry Accounting

In a healthcare organization, understanding assets and liabilities can impact the financial outcomes of a medical facility. Assets are defined as items owned by the facility. Liabilities are defined as items owed by the facility. **Net worth** is the difference between total assets and total liabilities. Depending on the legal structure, terms used for net worth include owner's equity, capital stock and retained earnings, net assets, and fund balance.

> ### Key Chapter Equation: Accounting
> The accounting equation is used regularly in the accounting field in double-entry accounting and can be written several different ways, such as:
> **Assets = Liabilities + Net worth**
> **Net worth = Assets – Liabilities**

Double-entry bookkeeping and accounting form the basis for all modern financial reporting. Every event that has a financial impact on the organization needs to be entered into the financial records. Under **double-entry accounting**, each financial event is recorded with a two-part entry. Each entry is self-balancing, with a **debit** and a **credit**. The use of these debits and credits is determined by the basic **accounting equation**, as shown in Figure 4-1.

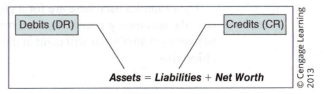

Figure 4-1 Basic Accounting Equation Used in Double-Entry Accounting

Assets, on the left side of the equation, are shown using **debits**. **Liabilities** and net worth, on the right side of the equation, are **credits**. Debits are frequently shown with the abbreviation *DR* and credits with the abbreviation *CR*. For the financial records as a whole to remain in balance, every individual entry must also be in balance with one or more debits equaling the amount of one or more credits. Double-entry accounting provides a method to verify that the financial records continue in balance. Table 4-1 shows the impact of an asset, liability, and net worth on a credit and debit when completing double-entry accounting.

Table 4-1: Impact of Assets on Credits and Debits

Assets	Credit	Debit
Assets Increase		X
Assets Decrease	X	
Liabilities Increase	X	
Liabilities Decrease		X
Revenue (Net worth Increases)	X	
Expense (Net worth Decreases)		X

At any time, a **trial balance** may be prepared. A trial balance is a listing of all of the current balances of all of the accounts in the financial system as of the date of the trial balance. A trial balance will always be prepared as part of the process of closing the books at the end of each fiscal year and will commonly be prepared on a monthly basis. When the total of all of the accounts with a debit balance equals the total of all of the accounts with a credit balance, the financial system is in balance. When the total does not balance, it becomes the responsibility of the accountant to review transactions from the date of the last trial balance to find and correct the posting error(s).

Types of Double-Entry Accounting Transactions

The key to proper bookkeeping and accounting is to post every financial event to the proper accounts. The following provides examples of common financial transactions and the proper way to record those using double-entry accounting. Each of the individual accounting transactions are combined with other transactions in the same account code during the course of the accounting period. The total activity in the account becomes the basis for the financial information in the balance sheet and income statement, discussed in following chapters.

The examples used here are for a physician's practice. As organizations increase in size, the accounting transactions become more complex. An itemized hospital bill for an overnight admission will contain much more information than the charge for a basic office visit.

Revenue Transaction

Example 4-1

Hadia Penna has an appointment to see the physician for a follow-up to her recent knee surgery. The bill for the office visit is $100, and she pays in cash that day. Cash is an asset of the business, carrying a debit balance. The cash received of $100 is an increase in an asset, so it will be posted as a debit to cash. The offsetting credit of $100 will be to a revenue account, Medical Services. **Revenues** are the funds that are earned by the physician's practice in providing medical services to patients. All revenues are recorded as credits in double-entry accounting.

The accounting entry for this transaction is shown in Figure 4-2.

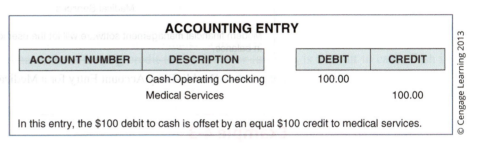

ACCOUNT NUMBER	DESCRIPTION	DEBIT	CREDIT
	Cash-Operating Checking	100.00	
	Medical Services		100.00

In this entry, the $100 debit to cash is offset by an equal $100 credit to medical services.

© Cengage Learning 2013

Figure 4-2 Double-Entry Account Entry for a Revenue Transaction

Accounts Receivable

Example 4-2

Charlie Kaminski comes into the practice for their annual physical examination. They have group health insurance that covers the full cost of preventive care based on the contract between the practice and the insurance company. The first accounting entry will record the medical service provided to Kaminski at the practice's standard billing rate of $250 and record an **accounts receivable** as an asset for the reimbursement due from the insurance company. When the insurance company pays the bill at the contract rate of $140, cash will be recorded as a debit, medical services revenue will be adjusted down by $110 to the contract amount, and the accounts receivable will be shown as fully paid.

The end result of these two accounting entries is that the medical facility has $140 in cash, and the net effect on medical services is a revenue balance of $140. There is no balance remaining in accounts receivable.

Accounts Payable

The previous examples deal with revenues earned by the practice. **Expenses** are the costs associated with earning those revenues. **Operating expenses** are the costs involved in running a business on a daily basis. Medical facilities will have a wide variety of operating expenses. Among these will be all of the costs related to the wages and benefits of the staffing of the practice, the purchase of medical and office supplies, and costs for utilities and maintenance. **Capital expenses** are the annual costs related to the decline in value over time of assets with a relatively long useful life.

The accounting entry for this transaction is shown in Figure 4-3.

When payments are made on the bank loan, three accounts are affected:

- The liability account for the bank loan is reduced by the amount paid on the principal balance of the loan.
- Interest paid on the bank loan is posted as an expense.
- Cash is reduced by the combined amount of the principal and interest paid on the loan.

Example 4-6

The medical practice of Dr. Ricca is located in a summer resort community. During the winter months, the number of patients seen decreases and the practice needs a short-term bank loan to be able to continue to meet its financial obligations. Dr. Ricca draws $10,000 from an existing bank line of credit. Figure 4-7 provides the account entry example for this transaction.

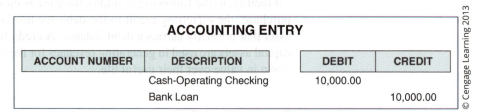

ACCOUNTING ENTRY			
ACCOUNT NUMBER	**DESCRIPTION**	**DEBIT**	**CREDIT**
	Cash-Operating Checking	10,000.00	
	Bank Loan		10,000.00

Figure 4-7 Account Entry for $10,000 Bank Loan in Example 4-6

Example 4-7

Interest due to the bank on the line of credit comes to $100 monthly on the outstanding balance of $10,000. As the business of the practice picks up as summer approaches, the Dr. Ricca medical practice is able to pay interest on the loan and begin to pay down the principal balance of the loan. In paying a bank loan, the interest and bank loan is a debit within the accounting entry, which is demonstrated in Figure 4-8.

ACCOUNTING ENTRY			
ACCOUNT NUMBER	**DESCRIPTION**	**DEBIT**	**CREDIT**
	Interest Expense	100.00	
	Bank Loan	1,000.00	
	Cash-Operating Checking		1,100.00

Figure 4-8 Payment Entry for Repaying Bank Loan

The account "Bank Loan" in this accounting entry started as the $10,000 liability account from Figure 4-7. The $1,000 payment on principal is posted as a debit, a reduction in the liability account, leaving a principal balance on the bank loan of $9,000.

The preceding examples illustrate common accounting transactions for any medical facility. The first step to properly account for any transaction is to identify the appropriate accounts to be used. All computerized financial management systems will have a **chart of accounts** that lists all of the account titles used in the system. The second step is to determine the dollar amount of the transaction. The third step is to assign debit and credit charges to the transaction. The fourth and final step is to ensure that the total of the debits on the entry equals the total of the credits.

As an example of this process, the bookkeeper for the physician practice is directed to pay the monthly electric bill of $250:

1. Step 1: Identify the accounts to be used. The chart of accounts includes an expense category for "utility expense." Cash held by the practice is used to pay the bill, so the second account affected is cash.

2. Step 2: Identify the amount. The bill for $250 will be paid in full.

3. Step 3: Assign debits and credits. Expenses carry a debit balance, so the debit on the entry will be to utility expense to show an increase in the expense account. Cash is an asset and assets carry a debit balance, so a reduction in the cash balance will require a credit.

4. Step 4: Ensure that debits and credits balance. Both are $250 and in balance.

This four-step process is used to account for all financial transactions of the medical facility. Repetitive transactions, such as positing revenues from patient visits, will quickly become automatic. Transactions that are more complicated or are used infrequently are more difficult and may require the assistance of the outside accountant used by the practice.

Comprehension Check 4.1

1. Dr. Martinez buys equipment and furniture for $120,000 on January 15, 2022, as well as computers for an additional $70,000 on January 15, 2022. Dr. Martinez pays cash for these items. However, for a new piece of medical equipment, Dr. Martinez takes a loan out for $190,000 on September 13, 2022. How would the journal transaction be recorded?

Date	Description	Debits	Credits

Knowledge Check

4.1

1. What is the basic accounting equation?

_____

_____

_____

2. On a monthly basis, the accountant for a nursing home runs a computer program that generates a trial balance. What is a trial balance, and what purpose does it serve?

_____

_____

_____

3. Elizabeth Bowen is self-employed and does not have healthcare insurance. She was injured in a fall at home and used her savings to pay the hospital bill for her knee operation. She was referred to Southwest Rehabilitation for therapy. Southwest charges $150 for each therapy session, and Ms. Bowen writes a check to pay for the services. Use the following form to show the accounting entry to record the service provided and payment received:

ACCOUNTING ENTRY			
ACCOUNT NUMBER	**DESCRIPTION**	**DEBIT**	**CREDIT**
	_____	_____	_____
	_____	_____	_____

© Cengage Learning 2013

4. Tahir Ahmad is also a therapy patient at Southwest Rehabilitation. Mr. Ahmad, however, is covered under a group insurance policy. The charge for therapy for both patients will be identical. Complete the following form to record the service provided to Mr. Ahmad and the billing to his insurance company.

ACCOUNTING ENTRY			
ACCOUNT NUMBER	**DESCRIPTION**	**DEBIT**	**CREDIT**
	_____	_____	_____
	_____	_____	_____
	_____	_____	_____

© Cengage Learning 2013

5. Mr. Ahmad's insurance company has a contract with Southwest that provides for a payment of $95 per therapy session. A check for that amount is received from the insurance company. Prepare the accounting entry to record the payment received and the necessary adjustments to both accounts receivable and medical services revenues:

continued

ACCOUNTING ENTRY

ACCOUNT NUMBER	DESCRIPTION	DEBIT	CREDIT

© Cengage Learning 2013

6. The maintenance supervisor at Central Hospital calls his supplier, Acme Industrial Supply, and orders a case of replacement furnace filters at a cost of $85. When the shipment is received, he inspects and signs the receiving ticket and reports the purchase to accounting. Prepare the following accounting entry to show this purchase:

ACCOUNTING ENTRY

ACCOUNT NUMBER	DESCRIPTION	DEBIT	CREDIT

© Cengage Learning 2013

7. At the end of the month, accounting receives an invoice from Acme Industrial for $85, compares the invoice to the approved receiving ticket, and issues a check to Acme. Prepare the following accounting entry for this payment:

ACCOUNTING ENTRY

ACCOUNT NUMBER	DESCRIPTION	DEBIT	CREDIT

© Cengage Learning 2013

8. Central Hospital uses computer software developed by Integrated Accounting Solutions to handle all of the basic accounting functions for the hospital. The software provider notifies the hospital that version 4.0 of the software is now available and that Integrated will no longer support older versions of the software. The charge for the software upgrade is $30,000, and Integrated will accept payment over 12 months with no interest. Central Hospital contracts and receives the software upgrade. Prepare the following accounting entry for this purchase:

ACCOUNTING ENTRY

ACCOUNT NUMBER	DESCRIPTION	DEBIT	CREDIT

© Cengage Learning 2013

continued

9. Peaceful Acres Nursing Home borrows $24,000 from the local bank to upgrade its kitchen facilities. The work is to be performed by a licensed contractor with payment due at completion of the work. Prepare the accounting entry to show the receipt of cash and obligation to the bank:

ACCOUNTING ENTRY

ACCOUNT NUMBER	DESCRIPTION		DEBIT	CREDIT

© Cengage Learning 2013

10. The loan agreement between the bank and Peaceful Acres calls for monthly payments of $2,000 to retire the loan over 12 months and interest on the unpaid balance paid monthly at the annual rate of 6 percent. Calculate the payment due at the end of the first month, and prepare the accounting entry to show the payment to the bank:

ACCOUNTING ENTRY

ACCOUNT NUMBER	DESCRIPTION		DEBIT	CREDIT

© Cengage Learning 2013

The Role of the Accountant in the Financial Process

"It is not easy to provide a concise definition of accounting since the word has a broad application within businesses and applications. The American Accounting Association defines accounting as follows: 'The process of identifying, measuring, and communicating economic information to permit informed judgments and decisions by the users of the information'."

(Tutor2U; http://tutor2u.net/business/accounts/intro_acctg)

The bookkeeping staff of a medical facility will be responsible for the recording of all financial transactions into the financial records. Medium- to large-size medical facilities will have professionally trained accountants on staff with the responsibility of reviewing and approving work performed by the bookkeeping staff, preparing financial statements and analysis for management, and ensuring that controls are in place to safeguard the assets of the organization. Smaller medical facilities will use an outside bookkeeping or accounting service to prepare financial statements and tax returns. Publicly held corporations and medical facilities operated by government agencies will be required to have an annual audit of their financial records. It is the responsibility of the outside auditors to ensure that the financial statements accurately reflect the financial position of the organization audited.

Computerized Accounting Systems in Health Care

"The first rule of any technology used in a business is that automation applied to an efficient operation will magnify the efficiency. The second is that automation applied to an inefficient operation will magnify the inefficiency."

(Bill Gates, founder, Microsoft; www.billgatesmicrosoft.com)

We live and work in the computer age. Ledgers and journals used to be handwritten in large books. Think of Bob Cratchit in *A Christmas Carol*, toiling by candlelight and using a quill pen to maintain account books. Today, accounting functions have been computerized, with sophisticated software programs handling everything from basic patient information, to bookkeeping functions, to preparing insurance claims, to billing patients for balances due.

In the computer software industry, the pricing of each unit of software is based on the volume of units sold.

QuickBooks Online uses double-entry accounting, which means each transaction or event changes two or more accounts in the ledger. Each of these changes involves a debit and a credit applied to one or more accounts. For most transactions, the entries of debits and credits are handled by QuickBooks Online.

Practice management systems (PMS) are comprehensive computer software programs designed specifically for medical offices. PMS supports a database function for all of the patient information, maintains schedules, files insurance claims, generates patient billings, and automatically updates the accounting records. Given the wide acceptance in the medical office community, these programs are available at an affordable cost.

As medical facilities grow larger, with increasingly complex programs tailored for a specific customer, the costs increase greatly. Software packages are available from outside vendors and are adapted for individual clients and then supported by a combination of vendor support and in-house information technology staffs.

The process of learning how a financial management system works is a manual one. Examples and review questions involve completing journal entries with handwritten account descriptions and amounts. Journal entries are totaled by hand to ensure debits and credits balance. In the work environment, financial management systems are automated. The following provides a conversion from manual to automated systems. In a manual accounting system:

1. In the current accounting period, business transactions such as posting revenues from providing medical services and recording cash received are analyzed and manually posted to handwritten journals. Journals maintained would include a cash receipts journal, a cash disbursements journal, and a revenue journal.

2. Individual entries from each of the journals are totaled, and summary totals from the journals are posted to the **general ledger**.

3. At the end of the current accounting period, a trial balance is prepared to ensure that the books are in balance.

4. Adjusting entries, such as depreciation of fixed assets for the current period and posting of prepaid expenses for the end of the current accounting period, are prepared and posted to the general ledger.

5. A worksheet is prepared and used for the preparation of the final trial balance.

6. The final trial balance is used to prepare financial statements for the current accounting period.

7. To prepare for the start of the new accounting cycle, journal entries are prepared and posted to close all revenue and expense accounts.

8. The final step in the cycle is the preparation of a post-closing trial balance. All revenue and expense accounts will have a zero balance, and the ending asset, liability, and equity account balances will become the beginning balances for the new cycle.

With a computerized accounting system, the following steps are used:

1. Each of the day-to-day business transactions are keyed into the appropriate computerized journal.

2. Summary totals from the journals are posted to the general ledger by the computer.

3. When prompted by the user, the computer will produce a trial balance.

4. At the end of the accounting period, journal entries will be drafted and keyed into the computer.

5. A final trial balance will be generated without the need for a worksheet.

6. The computer will automatically prepare and post closing entries to zero out revenue and expense accounts.

7. The computer will generate a post-closing trial balance.

The computerized accounting system is able to automatically perform many of the bookkeeping functions, such as totaling journals and posting the totals to the general ledger, more quickly and accurately than manual operations. What the computer is not able to do is tell the difference between a business transaction posted to the appropriate account and one that is not. If a hospital accounting clerk codes the purchase of medical supplies for the operating room to the account used for food purchases, the computer will accept the entry. Computerized accounting systems have safeguards built in to reduce error frequency. Vendor codes are linked to specific expense account numbers to avoid posting errors such as the example used here. These types of errors, when the dollar amounts are significant to the size of the operation, can adversely impact the accuracy of Medicare cost reports required from hospitals and the reliability of the internal budget to actual comparisons.

The position of the accountant continues to be needed in the computerized accounting environment. The process of analyzing transactions and ensuring that entries are posted to the proper accounts remains an important responsibility. Trial balances and financial statements need to be reviewed for accuracy and approved before reports are released. Computerized database and financial management systems eliminate much of the work that previously needed to be done by hand. However, these computerized systems never remove the need for basic management control of the process: competent employees need to be hired, trained, and motivated; supervisors need to review work performed by subordinates for accuracy; the financial statements that are the end output of the process need to be reviewed and approved; and software and work procedures need to be updated to meet changing facility needs and to meet new legal requirements.

Key Concepts

- Accounting is the language of business, and understanding this language is critical to the ability to understand and interpret financial statements.

- Double-entry accounting is based on the fundamental accounting equation: assets = liabilities + net worth. Every individual accounting entry must be self-balancing, with one or more *debits* equaling one or more *credits*.

- The role of the *bookkeeper* in the accounting system is to record transactions that impact the finances of the business. The *accountant* reviews and approves these entries, prepares financial statements, ensures that financial controls are in place and effective, and presents financial reports and analysis to top management.

- Computerized financial management systems have removed much of the labor-intensive work from the bookkeeping process. However, effective management controls need to be in place to ensure the accuracy of the financial records.

Accounting and the Financial Management Process

Key Terms

Accrual accounting
Cash accounting
Consistency
Financial accounting
Full disclosure
Generally accepted accounting principles (GAAP)
Going concern
Managerial accounting
Matching
Materiality
Stakeholders
Subsequent events

Chapter Objectives

After completing this chapter, readers should be able to:

- Illustrate the differences in the levels of accounting expertise among various sizes of healthcare facilities.

- Differentiate between financial accounting and managerial accounting.

- Explain the various stakeholders in the financing of health care.

- Identify generally accepted accounting principles (GAAP).

Chapter Glossary

Accrual accounting is the system of accounting that records revenues in the accounting period in which they are earned and expenses in the accounting period in which the resources are used.

Cash accounting is the system of accounting that records revenues in the accounting period in which cash payment is received and expenses in the accounting period when payment is made.

Consistency is the accounting policy requiring that once the proper accounting treatment for an issue has been determined, the same process should be applied for years.

Financial accounting is involved in the preparation of financial documents that are primarily intended for outside users.

Full disclosure is the principle that any events that may have an impact on the financial condition of the organization need to be disclosed in the annual financial report.

Generally accepted accounting principles (GAAP) are the basic standards and rules that accountants follow in recording financial transactions and reporting results.

Going concern concept is the accounting principle that values assets and liabilities of the business under the assumption that the medical facility will continue in business, with receivables being collected when due and payables paid from revenues of continuing business operations.

Managerial accounting is involved in the preparation of financial documents that are primarily intended for internal use within the organization.

Matching is the accounting principle that states that revenues are posted in the accounting period when services are provided and expenses are posted when resources are used.

Materiality is the accounting principle that requires that any accounting error that will have a significant impact on the financial statements of the business entity must be corrected.

Stakeholders in health care include all people and outside organizations that are directly impacted by the performance of healthcare facilities.

Subsequent events are actions of a material nature, occurring after the end of the financial reporting period but prior to the date of the accountant's report, that need to be disclosed in the annual financial report.

Introduction

The level of sophistication in accounting and financial management for healthcare organizations will generally depend on the size of the organization. A single physician practice will commonly employ a bookkeeper to prepare and mail account billings, pay the bills, and prepare the bank deposits. The work of the bookkeeper will be supplemented with the use of an outside accounting firm, hired to prepare the financial statements and tax returns. A hospital will have an in-house professional staff headed by the chief financial officer (CFO). Staffing may include professional accountants, a budget manager, and several accounting clerks to handle the bookkeeping functions. Risk management may be included within the responsibilities of the finance department. Audited financial statements are required for publicly held corporations and government agencies and are commonly used by other healthcare facilities. The financial statements are the responsibility of the in-house professional staff. Outside auditors are retained to review accounting activities and attest to the accuracy of the financial statements. Organization charts for a single physician's practice and a hospital's finance department in Figures 5-1 and 5-2 illustrate the differences in staffing.

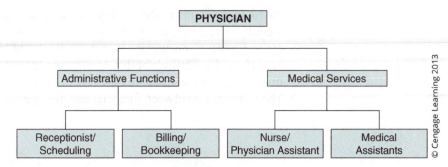

Figure 5-1 Single Physician Practice Office Structure

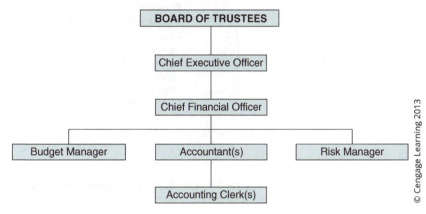

Figure 5-2 Example of a Hospital Finance Department

Financial Accounting and Managerial Accounting

The work of accountants in preparing financial reports and analyses is divided into two categories based on the users of the reports. **Financial accounting** is involved in the preparation of financial documents that are primarily intended for outside users. Examples of the types of reports that will be generated under the heading of financial accounting will include:

- Reports to governmental programs such as Medicare and Medicaid

- Reports to stockholders in publicly owned healthcare facilities

- Financial statements and budgets of governmental healthcare agencies to provide information to taxpayers

Managerial accounting is involved in the preparation of financial documents that are primarily intended for internal use. As the name implies, these reports are prepared to assist managers within the organization. Examples of the types of reports that will be generated under the heading of managerial accounting will include:

- Monthly budget-to-actual-expense reports for each operating unit of the facility

- Profitability forecasts

- Break-even analysis for adding new medical services

Many of the accounting reports generated by the finance department benefit both internal and external users. The annual balance sheet and income statements, discussed in upcoming chapters, provide valuable information to stockholders and taxpayers on the financial status of the facility and are also used by internal management staff to identify and address any problem areas in financial performance. Budget documents are important to management and are also used by banks and bond rating agencies to analyze the facility's ability to repay proposed debt. The professional staff in the finance department needs to be aware of the potential audience for the reports issued. The relationship between financial and managerial accounting is shown in Figure 5-3.

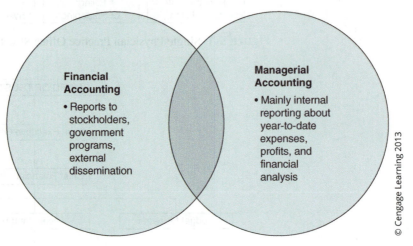

Figure 5-3 Overlapping Relationship Between Financial and Managerial Accounting

Stakeholders in Healthcare Finance

Stakeholders in the business of health care include all people and outside organizations that are directly impacted by the financial performance of individual healthcare facilities. Health care is much more than taking care of the medical needs of people; it is also about understanding the various influences on the business of health care. Stakeholders range from the individual investor looking to enjoy future profits from the purchase of stock, to the entry-level employee concerned that their job may be eliminated in a recession, to the retired couple who serve as volunteers in the local hospital and have made cash contributions to building a new cancer unit. These stakeholders will include the following:

- **Owners** and **partners** have an equity position in the facility. The value of their investment is directly tied to the profitability of the business.

- **Governing boards** have the stewardship function of ensuring that the facility uses financial resources to best meet the mission of the organization.

- **Stockholders** have their capital at risk through the purchase of stock in publicly traded healthcare corporations. If the corporation is profitable and the business is expanding, the stock price should increase, providing additional value to the stockholders. When the business is not doing well, the stock price will decline.

- **Bondholders** have invested funds in the healthcare facility with the expectation that interest payments will be received as promised and the principal invested will be returned at maturity of the bond.

- **Investment bankers and rating agencies** rely on financial information to assess the credit worthiness of the healthcare facility and to assist in raising capital funds.

- **Employees** have their and their families' livelihoods tied to the financial viability of their employer. Healthcare facilities that are doing well financially will tend to reward employees with pay raises and the opportunity for overtime and advancement. Facilities that are losing money from low patient census counts will attempt to balance the books with strategies such as call-offs, where employees are told not to report for scheduled shifts; pay freezes; and layoffs.

- **Managers** of work units in healthcare facilities are judged both for the professional competence of the work performed as well as for financial performance. Managers are assigned a budget and are expected to accomplish the mission of the work unit within those financial resources.

- **Customers** (patients, residents, or clients in healthcare organizations) can be seriously affected by the financial performance of healthcare facilities. For example, a doctor closes their practice and moves to a larger community where the financial opportunities are greater or a local hospital is forced to cut back on services provided when the revenues are not sufficient to support specialized services.

- **Creditors** are investing money in a healthcare facility from the time when goods are delivered or services provided until the facility makes payment. The creditor needs to be comfortable that payments will be made as promised. Banks and equipment leasing companies have much longer relationships with the facilities and base the decision to provide credit on their review of the financial documents of the facility.

- **Government** at the city, state, and federal levels all receive tax receipts from for-profit healthcare facilities. Information from the accounting system is used both to calculate the taxes and for the government to audit the accuracy of the taxes paid.

- **Taxpayers** own many healthcare facilities in this country, either in the form of public healthcare authorities or local governments own hospitals and health clinics. Taxpayers in the local communities where these healthcare facilities conduct their operations are ultimately responsible when facilities cannot meet operating costs and require government subsidies.

- **Benefactors** are individuals in local communities who donate their money and time to healthcare facilities.

Generally Accepted Accounting Principles

Generally accepted accounting principles (GAAP) are the basic standards and rules that accountants follow in recording financial transactions and reporting results. GAAP govern the form and content of the financial statements of an entity and encompass the conventions, rules, and procedures necessary to define accepted accounting practice at a particular time. They include not only broad guidelines of general application but also detailed practices and procedures. The primary authoritative body on the application of GAAP to state and local governments is the Governmental Accounting Standards Board.

GAAP have been developed and codified under the direction of the Financial Accounting Standards Board (FASB) and accepted by the American Institute of Certified Public Accountants (AICPA) to provide for consistency in financial reporting. Further information on these organizations may be found on their respective websites: *www.fasb.org* and *www.aicpa.org*. The AICPA performs similar roles for professional accountants as the American Medical Association (AMA) does for physicians, promoting the profession and providing educational programs to allow practitioners to keep their skills current.

In summary, GAAP are standards developed by the profession to ensure that readers of financial statements are provided with a complete and accurate assessment of the financial status of a business. Accounting is more art than science. The application of the rules of GAAP requires the use of estimates and judgments by professional accountants in the reporting of financial results.

BOX 5-1 GAAP Rules and Standards

- Going concern concept
- Matching
- Consistency
- Materiality
- Full disclosure

Going Concern Concept

Accountants will value the assets and liabilities of the medical facility under the assumption that the facility will continue in business. The assets are the items of value, such as cash, inventory, balances owed by patients and insurance companies for medical services provided, and building and equipment owned by the medical facility. For a **going concern**, these assets are traditionally valued at cost. When a business fails, the amount of cash that may be realized in the sale of the assets may well be far less than the value carried on the books of the business. Medical facilities may close for several reasons. A community hospital in a small town may be forced to close when the patient base is not sufficient to cover the costs of staying in business. A physician practice may close on the retirement of the physician. Liabilities are the unpaid financial obligations of the medical facility, such as normal bills for goods and services received that have not yet been paid and any bank loans or equipment loans outstanding. For a going concern, the assumption is made that the obligations will be paid as they come due. Therefore, the assets and liabilities of the medical facility are carried on the financial records at full value. When a business fails, funds may or may not be available to cover these debts.

Comprehension Check 5.1

Within a healthcare facility, there are several assets and liabilities that are used daily. In the following list, identify the assets and liabilities.

Long-term loan

Equipment

Cash

Rent

Medical gloves

Inventory

Matching

Individuals are familiar with **cash accounting** in their state and federal income taxes. Pay earned during the last few days in December may well be paid in the first paycheck received in January, with taxes withheld and reported in January. An individual may pledge a donation to their church in December 2010 but not pay by check until the following month, January 2011. The donation will then be reported in the individual's 2011 federal tax form 1040. In **accrual accounting**, the accepted accounting standard for businesses, revenues are posted when they are earned, and expenses are posted as the resources are used. Under accrual accounting, pay earned by employees during the last few days in December and paid in January will be treated as a December expense. A business that pledges a donation to a local charity in December and sends the check in January will record the donation on the books for December when the pledge is made. Accrual accounting provides **matching**, allowing for both revenues and expenses to be posted in the proper accounting period and for costs incurred in providing services to be matched against the revenues generated by those services. This differs from cash accounting in business, where revenues are not posted until cash payment has been received and expenses are not posted until the bills have been paid.

Comprehension Check 5.2

An employee at Heart Felt Medical Facility receives a $2,000 bonus based on a having outstanding patient satisfaction reviews in December 2020. The bonus is not paid until January 2021. Based on the matching principle, what year should the bonus be recorded?

Example 5-1

Dr. Zawba runs a single-physician practice, and the books are maintained on a calendar year. In the month of December, the practice sees several patients covered by group medical insurance. Even though insurance payments will not be received until January, the revenues will be booked in December and the amount owed by insurance shown as an account receivable. Many of the expenses of running the practice for the month of December will not be paid until January, such as payment for December utilities and shipments of medical supplies ordered and received in December. These expenses will be booked in the month of December and the amount owed by the practice shown as accounts payable.

One of the most common applications of the principle of matching is in the accounting treatment of the purchase of a piece of equipment, showing its decline in value through an annual charge for depreciation as it is used over the years.

To determine the annual depreciation on each asset, the straight-line method can be used to calculate accumulated depreciation.

Key Chapter Equation: Straight-Line Method

The straight-line equation is:
Purchase Price-Salvage Value/Years in Useful Life

A dialysis machine costs $100,000 and is expected to be in use for a period of 10 years from the date of acquisition. After 10 years, it will be worn out and disposed of with no resale value. Each year for 10 years, one-tenth of the cost, or $10,000, is removed from the original value and shown as an annual operating expense of the medical facility. At the end of 10 years, the book value has been reduced to zero through accumulated depreciation. The annual operating results of the medical practice appropriately match the costs of the equipment wearing out against revenues earned from medical services provided that year.

Consistency

Once the accountant and the medical facility have agreed on the proper accounting treatment of financial events, the principle of **consistency** states that the same method of treatment should be used in future years. When a piece of capital equipment has been purchased and the useful life projected to be 10 years, the useful life should not be arbitrarily changed to 5 years in the following accounting year.

Materiality

In recording the thousands of individual transactions that occur over the course of a fiscal year, errors will happen. The principle of **materiality** requires any errors that have a significant impact on the accuracy of the financial statements to be corrected. When conducting an audit, auditors will closely review all major areas of financial activity, such as the purchase of major capital equipment or construction activity. Auditors will also select a random sample of routine financial activity for review. A full review of all transactions, termed a **forensic audit**, is cost prohibitive for a routine audit and is only used in audits to determine fraud or mismanagement. What is a material error for a small medical facility may not be a material error for a large organization. In actual practice, implementing materiality is based on the informed judgment of professional accountants and auditors. Review Case Study 5-1.

Case Study 5-1

Longview Regional Hospital has established a set of financial controls that include making department supervisors responsible for operating their functions within the approved budget. Outside auditors are hired by Longview to review financial activity each year. A sampling of financial transactions by the auditors revealed two errors:

1. Early in the fiscal year, Longview contracted with a new landscape maintenance company at a monthly contract rate of $1,500. Personnel in the accounting department set up a vendor account for the new landscape company and properly coded the payment to an account titled "contractual services." An error was made in coding the charge to the housekeeping department rather than the facilities department. Total charges recorded during the year totaled more than $10,000.

2. The local office supply company provides products used by various departments of the hospital. A purchase in the amount of $95 was properly approved and paid but was charged to the wrong department.

You are the auditor who was given the Longview Regional Hospital assignment and discovered the preceding two errors in the financial records. Errors that are considered material should be corrected, and errors considered minor do not require correction. What recommendations would you make to the accounting staff at Longview?

The first error in Case Study 5-1, the contract for landscape maintenance, was considered by the auditor to be a material error. The housekeeping department was over budget for the year due to the error, and improper postings would continue into the new fiscal year unless corrected. The auditor brought the issue to the attention of the hospital's accounting manager and requested that the error be corrected. The second error was considered to be minor. The auditor noted the error in their work papers but took no further action.

Full Disclosure

Any events that may have an impact on the financial condition of the organization need to be disclosed in the annual financial report; this is called **full disclosure**. This includes any events that may occur from the end of the accounting year to the date that the financial reports are dated and released. A pharmaceutical research company uses a calendar year as its accounting year. In January, after the end of the accounting year but prior to the date of the financial reports prepared by the outside accountant, the U.S. Food and Drug Administration refuses to approve a new drug developed by the company. This event will have an obvious negative impact on the financial health of the company and must be disclosed as part of the financial statements of the company. Actions that occur after the end of the accounting period that are material and need to be disclosed are referred to as **subsequent events**.

Knowledge Check 5.1

1. Describe the differences between financial accounting and managerial accounting.

_____

_____

_____

2. What are generally accepted accounting principles (GAAP)?

_____

_____

_____

3. Define the concept of stakeholder. Who are the major stakeholders in health care?

_____

_____

_____

4. Explain the accounting principle of the going concern concept.

_____

_____

_____

5. Matching is the accounting principle that states that, in accrual accounting, revenues are posted based on the date when they are earned, and expenses are posted as costs are incurred and resources used. How does this differ from cash accounting, and what types of adjustments must be made by the accountant at year-end under accrual accounting?

_____

_____

_____

6. Provide an example of the use of the accounting principle of consistency.

_____

_____

_____

7. Explain the accounting principle of materiality.

_____

_____

_____

8. Northridge Hospital is an investor-owned, for-profit hospital. The hospital maintains its financial records on a calendar year. In February, after the end of the latest fiscal year but prior to the date of the release of its financial statements for the year, Northridge suffers a fire that causes the closure of one of the patient wings. Repairs will take a minimum of 90 days to complete to allow the wing to be reopened. Which accounting principle requires that this event be disclosed in the hospital's financial statements?

_____

_____

_____

Key Concepts

- Financial accounting is the preparation of financial and accounting reports generally intended for outside users. Managerial accounting is the preparation of financial and accounting reports generally intended for users internal to the healthcare organization.

- Stakeholders in health care are all the individuals and outside organizations that are directly impacted by the healthcare facility. In addition to the patients who use the facility, these will include owners and partners, governing boards, stockholders and bondholders, employees, suppliers and creditors, government, and taxpayers and benefactors.

- Generally accepted accounting principles (GAAP) are the basic standards and rules used by accountants in the preparation of financial statements. Important standards include:

  - Going concern concept
  - Matching
  - Consistency
  - Materiality
  - Full disclosure

The Balance Sheet

Key Terms

Accumulated depreciation
Balance sheet
Book value
Contra account
Current assets
Current liabilities
Depreciation expense
Equity ownership
Fiscal year
Goodwill
Intangible assets
Non-current assets
Non-current liabilities
Salvage value
Straight-line method
Tangible assets

Chapter Objectives

After completing this chapter, readers should be able to:

- Explain the types of accounting items categorized as assets, including the distinction between current and non-current assets.

- Explain the concept and application of depreciation and accumulated depreciation.

- Classify liability accounts, including the distinction between current and non-current liabilities.

- Describe how net worth is calculated and the different titles used for net worth, based on the legal structure of the business.

Chapter Glossary

Accumulated depreciation is the total value of the annual charges for **depreciation** (see later definition) of an asset since that asset was placed into service.

The **balance sheet** displays all the items owned by the business, all debts that are owed, and the book value of the business at a certain point in time.

The **book value** of an asset is the value asset on the financial statements representing the original cost of the asset less the accumulated depreciation recorded since the asset was placed in use.

A **contra account** is used to reduce the value of an asset account by the estimated loss in value of the asset. Contra accounts are most commonly used to record the estimated value of uncollectible accounts receivable and to record accumulated depreciation of capital assets.

Current assets are those assets that will be used by the business within a 12-month period.

Current liabilities are amounts owed by a business that are expected to be paid during the next 12 months.

Depreciation expense is the measurement of loss in value of a capital asset, charged annually, as it ages or is used up during business.

Equity ownership, also known as net worth, is the book value of the business for the owner, partner, or shareholders.

Fiscal year is a consecutive 12-month period chosen by the business to report financial operations.

Goodwill is a business asset recognized when a business is purchased for an amount greater than the total book value of the assets purchased.

Intangible assets are assets of value to the business, but do not have a physical existence, such as patents, copyrights, goodwill, and investment in research and development.

Non-current assets are those assets that will be used by the business for a period greater than 1 year.

Non-current liabilities are amounts owed by a business that are expected to be paid at a date in the future more than 12 months away.

Salvage value is an accounting term referring to the amount of money expected to be realized from the sale of used assets, normally furniture and equipment.

Straight-line method is a method used to calculate accumulated depreciation. The formula is: (Purchase Price − Salvage Value/Years in Useful Life).

Tangible assets are those assets owned by the business, such as buildings and equipment, that have a physical existence.

Introduction

The **balance sheet** is a snapshot of the financial status of a healthcare facility at a certain point in time. While a balance sheet may be prepared as of any date, the date of the year-end balance sheet represents the ending date of the **fiscal year** of the business, the consecutive 12-month period that the business has chosen to report financial results. Businesses may choose a fiscal year that corresponds to the normal annual cycle of the type of business it is engaged in. Most healthcare facilities will follow a calendar year as their fiscal year. The most common selections are January 1st through December 31st, July 1st through June 30th, or October 1st through September 30th. A different fiscal year may be used so that the year-end work by their outside accountant is a slower time of year than the end of the calendar year, when accountants are busy preparing personal income taxes and financial reports of businesses that operate on a calendar year.

The balance sheet shows the assets of the business ("what is owned"), liabilities ("what is owed"), and the difference between the two. As the name implies, the two sides of the balance sheet will always remain in balance when the statement is properly prepared.

The difference between the two represents the equity ownership of the business. Equity ownership, also referred to as net worth, is the book value of the business for the owner, partner, or shareholders. **Equity ownership** within a medical facility is based on assets and liabilities. To determine the equity within a medical facility, the Equity Ownership Equation can be used.

Key Chapter Equation: Accounting

The Accounting Equation can be written in various ways. The two equations that you will see most often in accounting are:

Owner's Equity = Assets − Liabilities
Assets = Liabilities + Owner's Equity

Refer to Figure 6-1 for an example balance sheet.

Lakeview Medical Clinic
Balance Sheet
December 31, 20XX

ASSETS			LIABILITIES & NET WORTH	
Current Assets	**Debit**	**Credit**	**Current Liabilities**	
Cash & Cash Equivalents		$15,000	Accounts Payable	$5,200
Short-Term Investments		$25,000	Accrued Expenses	$7,400
Accounts Receivable	$75,000		Current Portion of	
Less: Allowance Uncollectible Accts	−$1,500	$73,500	Long-Term Debt	$37,800
Supplies		$2,000		
Prepaid Expenses		$4,000	**Total Current Liabilities**	$50,400
Total Current Assets		$119,500	**Non-Current Liabilities**	
Non-Current Assets			Long-Term Debt:	
			Net of Current Portion	$250,000
Land		$100,000		
Buildings	$350,000		**Total Non-Current Liabilities**	$250,000
Furniture & Equipment	$175,000			
Less: Accumulated Depreciation	−$75,000	$450,000	**NET WORTH**	
Other Assets		$50,000		
			Owners' Equity	$419,100
Total Non-Current Assets		$600,000		
			TOTAL LIABILITIES &	
TOTAL ASSETS		$719,500	**NET WORTH**	$719,500

© Cengage Learning 2013

Figure 6-1 Lakeview Medical Clinic Balance Sheet

Example 6-1

Lakeview Medical Clinic is a freestanding medical services provider. It is legally organized as a sole proprietorship under the ownership of Dr. Bowers. The medical clinic provides family medical services, treating many families covered by group health insurance and senior citizens covered by Medicare. The clinic owns the land and building where the practice is located and owns the medical equipment used by the practice. The property is secured by a mortgage negotiated through the local bank, with monthly payments of principal and interest paid on the loan. This monthly payment to the bank comprises two parts: principal, which is repayment on the balance of the loan, and interest, which is an expense for the time value of money cost of the use of the bank's money. Lakeview Medical has also financed several pieces of expensive durable medical equipment with loans from the supplier of the equipment; the facility is making monthly payments on those loans. The practice has been successful over the several years that Dr. Bowers has overseen the practice. Dr. Bowers has built a significant equity in the business, $419,100 as of December 31, 20XX, as shown in the balance sheet for the practice in Figure 6-1. Equity represents Dr. Bowers' ownership stake in the business, the difference between total assets and total liabilities. In this manner, the two sides of the balance sheet continue to be equal, with the total of the assets of the business equal to the combination of the total liabilities and net worth.

Assets

Assets are items with a measurable financial value that are owned by the business. Assets are divided into current and non-current assets. **Current assets** are those assets that can reasonably be expected to be used by the business within a 12-month period. **Non-current assets** are those assets that will be used by the business for a period greater than 12 months.

Current Assets

Assets were previously defined as those items that are owned by the business. Current assets include:

- Cash balances
- Short-term investments
- Accounts receivable
- Supplies
- Any prepaid expenses
- Inventory

Figure 6-2 provides an example of these potential current assets.

Cash & Cash Equivalents

Cash & cash equivalents include several items either held in cash or readily converted to cash:

- Petty cash is the small cash balance held in the bookkeeping office to pay minor expenses such as postage and minor office supplies purchases.
- The cash balance in the cash drawer is used to make change for patients and clients paying their bills in cash.
- The operating checking account for the medical facility is used both for the deposit of funds received by the facility for services provided and to pay the bills of the facility as they become due. In addition to the operating checking account, many facilities will choose to have a separate checking account for payroll activities.
- Short-term investments will include items such as money market accounts used to generate additional interest income and any short-term investments, such as a 30-day certificate of deposit or a 91-day U.S. treasury bill. **Liquidity** means the degree to which an asset can be converted to cash.

Lakeview Medical Clinic
Balance Sheet
December 31, 20XX

> Current assets are those assets that will be used by the business within a 12-month period.

ASSETS				LIABILITIES & NET WORTH	
Current Assets	**Debit**	**Credit**		**Current Liabilities**	
Cash & Cash Equivalents		$15,000		Accounts Payable	$5,200
Short-Term Investments		$25,000		Accrued Expenses	$7,400
Accounts Receivable	$75,000			Current Portion of	
Less: Allowance Uncollectible Accts	−$1,500	$73,500		Long-Term Debt	$37,800
Supplies		$2,000			
Prepaid Expenses		$4,000		**Total Current Liabilities**	$50,400
Total Current Assets		$119,500		**Non-Current Liabilities**	
Non-Current Assets				Long-Term Debt:	
				Net of Current Portion	$250,000
Land		$100,000			
Buildings	$350,000			**Total Non-Current Liabilities**	$250,000
Furniture & Equipment	$175,000				
Less: Accumulated Depreciation	−$75,000	$450,000		**NET WORTH**	
Other Assets		$50,000			
				Owners' Equity	$419,100
Total Non-Current Assets		$600,000			
				TOTAL LIABILITIES &	
TOTAL ASSETS		**$719,500**		**NET WORTH**	**$719,500**

© Cengage Learning 2013

Figure 6-2 Lakeview Medical Clinic Current Assets on the Balance Sheet

Short-Term Investments

Short-term investments include any investments made by the business in securities that will mature in less than 12 months. The term **securities** will include investments made by the business in bank certificates of deposit, stocks that are actively traded on major stock exchanges, and bonds issued by corporations of government agencies. To be classified as short-term investments, they must have a maturity date of less than 12 months. The maturity date of a security is the date when the amount invested in the security is returned to the owner with interest.

Accounts Receivable

Accounts receivable are funds due for medical services that were not paid in cash at the time of service. Fifty years ago, medicine was a cash business. Managing the funds due from third parties has now become an important function of the financial accounting process for medical facilities. With the rise of group health insurance plans for employed adults and their dependents and Medicare for senior citizens more payments are made through accounts receivable. The Centers for Medicare & Medicaid Services (CMS) is the single largest payer for healthcare in the United States. Nearly 90 million Americans rely on healthcare benefits through Medicare, Medicaid, and the State Children's Health Insurance Program (SCHIP).

https://www.cms.gov/blog/creating-roadmap-end-covid-19-public-health-emergency

The balance sheet item for accounts receivable will show the total balance for unpaid medical services as of the balance sheet date. Not all this money will end up being collected. Patients die or move away. Claims may be rejected by insurance companies or government providers that for various reasons cannot be corrected and resubmitted for payment. Figure 6-3 illustrates the revenue claim cycle. The revenue claim cycle tracks the patient from their visit all the way through the claim submission process.

will appear on the balance sheet. For companies such as providers of durable medical equipment, a major portion of the assets of the company may be invested in their inventory held for sales to medical facilities or direct to patients. Inventory is taken as of the last day of the fiscal year and valued by the accounting staff for financial statement presentation.

Non-Current Assets

Non-current assets are those assets that will be used in the business for a period greater than 12 months.

Non-current assets include:

- Land
- Buildings
- Furniture
- Equipment
- Other Assets

All medical facilities will have some assets with a reasonably long useful life, such as medical equipment and furniture. Businesses that own their own facility will have balance sheet items for land and buildings. Some medical facilities will have other non-current assets such as their investment in computer hardware and software, improvements to leased property, and goodwill. All these non-current assets, except for land, will decline in value over time as a function of usage or obsolescence. The annual reduction in value is accounted for with the use of a charge for depreciation. The annual charges for depreciation are accumulated over the years that the asset is owned until the value of the asset is reduced to zero. Figure 6-4 highlights non-current assets on the Lakeview Medical Clinic balance sheet from Figure 6-1.

Lakeview Medical Clinic
Balance Sheet
December 31, 20XX

ASSETS			LIABILITIES & NET WORTH	
Current Assets	Debit	Credit	**Current Liabilities**	
Cash & Cash Equivalents		$15,000	Accounts Payable	$5,200
Short-Term Investments		$25,000	Accrued Expenses	$7,400
Accounts Receivable	$75,000		Current Portion of	
Less: Allowance Uncollectible Accts	−$1,500	$73,500	Long-Term Debt	$37,800
Supplies		$2,000		
Prepaid Expenses		$4,000	**Total Current Liabilities**	$50,400
Total Current Assets		$119,500	**Non-Current Liabilities**	
Non-Current Assets				
			Long-Term Debt:	
Land		$100,000	Net of Current Portion	$250,000
Buildings	$350,000			
Furniture & Equipment	$175,000		**Total Non-Current Liabilities**	$250,000
Less: Accumulated Depreciation	−$75,000	$450,000	**NET WORTH**	
Other Assets		$50,000		
			Owners' Equity	$419,100
Total Non-Current Assets		$600,000		
			TOTAL LIABILITIES &	
TOTAL ASSETS		**$719,500**	**NET WORTH**	**$719,500**

*Non-current assets are those assets that will be used by the business for a period of time greater than 1 year.

© Cengage Learning 2013

Figure 6-4 Lakeview Medical Clinic Non-Current Assets on the Balance Sheet

Capital Assets

Capital assets are the items owned by the business, are used in the performance of the business, and have a useful life of greater than 1 year. The following types of items would be included under the heading of capital assets: land, buildings, durable medical equipment, furniture, computer hardware and software, and improvements to leased property. This listing includes the traditional items of capital assets that would be owned by a medical facility.

Other types of businesses will have additional capital assets on their financial records:

- **Goodwill** is created as an asset when a business is sold for an amount greater than the value of the assets purchased. The new owner agrees to pay a higher price under the premise that customers or patients will continue to do business there, generating profits for the new owner. There are several ways a goodwill asset can be utilized. A goodwill asset would be account receivables, customer lists, and prescription files provided to the new owner by the seller.

Example 6-2 helps explain the concept of goodwill.

Example 6-2

John Dillon, owner of Dillon's Pharmacy, is retiring and agrees to sell the business to Betty Spayde for $340,000. Ms. Spayde already owns and operates a pharmacy in the community, and the new location will be operated as part of her business. Dillon's Pharmacy leases space on Main Street. The packaging, handheld devices for order entry, refrigerators for storing medicine, and automatic dispensing machines are valued at $200,000, and business fixtures such as shelving, mirrors, locks, and handles are valued at $45,000. The balance of the purchase price, $95,000, is for goodwill.

- **Research and development costs** are the investments made by pharmaceutical companies in developing new drugs. These costs will be recovered from revenues from sales of the new drugs.

Capital assets are also classified as tangible or intangible, based on the physical nature of the asset. **Tangible assets** are those assets owned by the business, such as buildings and equipment that have a physical existence. **Intangible assets** are assets of value to the business, but do not have a physical existence, such as patents, copyrights, goodwill, and investment in research and development. Figure 6-5 shows how noncurrent assets can fall under three categories: tangible assets, intangible assets, and natural resources.

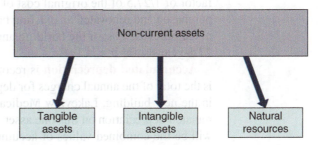

Figure 6-5 Non-Current Assets

Not all businesses will use all categories of non-current assets. Again, referring to Figure 6-1, Lakeview Medical does not have a significant investment in computer hardware and software and does not have improvements to leased property. Assets owned by Lakeview Medical that do not fit into the categories for land, buildings, or furniture and equipment are shown as **other assets** in this example.

Land

Land is recorded on the balance sheet at the cost basis of an undeveloped piece of real estate. Since land does not become worn out or obsolete, it stays on the books of the business at its original cost. The value of the land may increase or decrease due to general economic conditions, but accounting principles require that the value of the land for financial statement purposes continue at the original purchase price. In the example of Lakeview Medical Clinic, the decision was made several years ago to move from rental office space. Lakeview purchased a vacant parcel zoned for medical offices for $100,000 and contracted for the construction of the clinic. If Lakeview had purchased an existing building and land as a combined purchase, the accounting treatment of the value of the land becomes more subjective. The accountant for the clinic, working with the real-estate professionals involved in the purchase, would use available information on land values to assign a value to the land portion of the purchase and record that amount on the balance sheet.

Buildings

Buildings are assets with a long useful life that will reduce in value over time from age and obsolescence. There are tax benefits for buildings to be owned by the physician or partners as individuals and lease the building to the practice. However, specific factors must be met.

The IRS lists the factors required to meet the depreciation requirements.

- It must be property owned.

- It must be used in a business or income-producing activity.

- It must have a determinable useful life.

- It must be expected to last more than 1 year.

https://www.irs.gov/publications/p946#en_US_2020_publink100070018

In the Lakeview Medical Center example, Lakeview Medical owns the land and building. Accounting uses **depreciation expense** to measure the loss in value over time. For example, Lakeview Medical contracted for the construction of a new medical clinic in the amount of $350,000. Lakeview Medical's accountant has recommended a useful life for the building of 27.5 years, a standard established by the Internal Revenue Service. At the end of that period, the building is assumed to be obsolete and have no remaining value. To record this periodic reduction in value, an annual charge for depreciation will be posted on the accounting records using the factor of 1/27.5 of the original cost of $350,000, or $12,727. Had Lakeview Medical purchased and renovated an existing building, the cost of renovations would be added to the purchase cost of the building and the combined total depreciated over the same 27.5-year useful life.

Accumulated depreciation is recorded for every asset owned by the business and is the total of the annual charges for depreciation to each individual asset. After 3 years in the new building, Lakeview Medical will have $38,181 (3 times $12,727) in accumulated depreciation on this one asset. Accumulated depreciation on the balance sheet will be the combined values of accumulated depreciation on all depreciable assets of the clinic.

Furniture and Equipment

Furniture and equipment represent the total value of assets purchased for use in the business with more than minimal value and a relatively long useful life. Minor purchases, such as staplers and stethoscopes, will be treated as regular business expenses. Under Medicare regulations, furniture and equipment will include all assets purchased for the business with an original cost of $2,500 or more and a useful life of longer than 1 year. Office furniture and pieces of durable medical equipment will qualify as furniture and equipment.

// Comprehension Check 6.1

Dr. Swazy is opening a new dental practice. She is trying to organize her balance sheet to allow for current and non-current assets for her dental office. In the following list, identify the current (C) and non-current (NC) assets within Dr. Swazy's practice.

Patient dental chair

X-ray equipment

Sterilization equipment

Fax machines

Plastic cups

Surgical gloves

Office desks

Cabinetry

Dental operatory lights

Computers

Dental office building

Land

Accounts receivable

Short-term loan (8 months) on teeth-whitening machine

Protective masks

Depreciation Expense

Depreciation expense is the measurement of loss in value of a capital asset, charged annually, as it ages or is used up during business. Every individual asset that qualifies for accounting treatment as furniture and equipment is recorded at its cost. The cost of each asset will include the purchase price plus any related expenses, such as delivery and set-up costs. This becomes the initial **book value** of that asset. A medical facility makes the decision that top-of-the-line medical equipment will be purchased and will be sold for salvage value before it becomes seriously worn or outmoded. **Salvage value** is an accounting term referring to the amount of money that is expected to be realized from the sale of used equipment. In the new building, each examination room is equipped with a new examination table, purchased at a cost of $2,500 each. The facility makes the decision that these assets will be used for only 5 years then sold with a remaining salvage value of $500 each.

To determine the annual depreciation on each asset, the **straight-line method** can be used to calculate accumulated depreciation.

Key Chapter Equation: Straight-Line Method

The straight-line equation is:
Purchase Price − Salvage Value/Years in Useful Life

Each examination table will then have an annual charge for depreciation of $400 ($2,500 minus $500 divided by 5). The accounting entry to record the annual charge for depreciation on this asset is demonstrated in Figure 6-6.

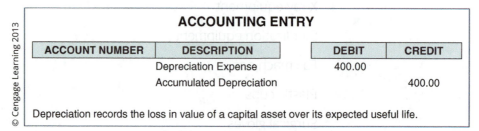

© Cengage Learning 2013

ACCOUNTING ENTRY			
ACCOUNT NUMBER	**DESCRIPTION**	**DEBIT**	**CREDIT**
	Depreciation Expense	400.00	
	Accumulated Depreciation		400.00

Depreciation records the loss in value of a capital asset over its expected useful life.

Figure 6-6 Accounting Entry for Depreciation of an Asset

Depreciation for the first year of ownership of an asset is based on the amount of time during the fiscal year that the asset was in service. An asset purchased and placed in service at the start of a fiscal year would have a full year's depreciation in the first year. An asset purchased and placed in service in the middle of a fiscal year would have only one-half of a full year's depreciation charged in the first year. Depreciation is an estimate, based on projections of useful life and salvage value. The book value of each asset is reduced by each year's charge for depreciation.

Accumulated depreciation is the total of the annual charges for depreciation for each individual asset. In the examination table example, the purchase price for each table was $2,500. At the end of the first year, the net book value of each examination table is $2,100 ($2,500 minus $400). Depreciation expense in the second year of use is an additional $400. The accumulated depreciation on this asset is then $800 ($400 annually for 2 years). The net book value of the asset at the end of the second year is then $1,700 ($2,500 less accumulated depreciation of $800).

When an asset is disposed of, both the original cost of the asset and the accumulated depreciation for the asset are removed from the financial records. Any money received from the sale of the used asset is recorded, and the financial records are balanced with an entry to a miscellaneous revenue or expense account. Continuing with the example of the examination tables, each table is sold after 5 years of use. After 5 years, each table has accumulated depreciation of $2,000 ($400 annually for 5 years). The net asset value is now $500 ($2,500 initial cost less $2,000 in accumulated depreciation). The table is then sold for $600. The $100 difference between cash received for the table and the net asset value of $500 is posted to the financial records as miscellaneous revenue. If the table had been sold for only $400, the $100 loss would be posted as a miscellaneous expense. Table 6-2 demonstrates the depreciation for 5 years within a table based on years.

Accumulated depreciation is the total charges for depreciation for each asset. If an examination table was purchased for $2,500 in the year 2019, the net book value of each examination table would be $2,100 at the end of the first year. The Purchase Price (Asset Cost) of $2,500 – Net Book Value $2,100 = $400

Table 6-2 Depreciation for Medical Equipment

Year	Asset Cost ($)	Yearly Depreciation ($)	Accumulated Depreciation ($)	Net Book Value ($)
2019	2,500	400	400	2,100
2020	2,500	400	800	1,700
2021	2,500	400	1,200	1,300
2022	2,500	400	1,600	900
2023	2,500	400	2,000	500

Depreciation in the examples used here is the logical process of writing off the value of an asset over its useful life. In the real world, depreciation becomes much more complicated. Depreciation is an expense, and total expenses of a business are offset against total revenues to determine the net income (profitability) and tax liability of a business. When expenses increase, taxable net income is reduced and taxes go down. When a business can write down the value of assets quicker through accelerated depreciation, total expenses are higher and taxable income is reduced. Tax laws provide a legal means for increasing the charge for depreciation of an asset during the early years of ownership, providing a stimulus to the economy by encouraging businesses to invest in new infrastructure. Smaller medical facilities will normally rely on the expertise of outside accountants to determine the most favorable tax treatment for depreciation of assets.

Comprehension Check 6.2

Dr. Lahayla paid $6,598 for a patient chair. She decided when purchasing the chair that she would sell the patient chair for salvage value before it becomes worn out. She plans to use the dental chair for 10 years and sell the chair for $1,000. To determine the annual depreciation on each asset, the straight-line method can be used to calculate accumulated depreciation. Calculate the annual depreciation. What would the accumulated depreciation be for 5 years?

Key Chapter Equation: Straight-Line Method

The straight-line equation is:
Purchase Price – Salvage Value/Years in Useful Life

Other Assets

Other assets is a category used to account for any items of value owned by the business that are not appropriately recorded in any other part of the balance sheet. Some businesses will have other assets that, similar to the loss in value over time of buildings and equipment, will decline annually in value. Examples of these types of assets would be costs to issue bonds and goodwill. Goodwill, discussed earlier, is recognized on the balance sheet when a business entity is purchased for an amount greater than the book value of the assets purchased. The decline in value of these assets is recognized with an annual charge for **amortization**. Depreciation is the periodic reduction in value of tangible assets; amortization is the periodic reduction in value of intangible assets. Bond issuance costs are a total of all the expenses related to selling bonds, such as outside attorney fees, rating agency fees, and the costs of printing bond prospectuses. These bond issuance costs will be amortized over the life of the bonds, and goodwill will be amortized over a reasonable period as the new ownership of the business becomes established in the marketplace.

Knowledge Check

6.1

1. Which of the following is NOT a current asset?
   A. Business checking account
   B. Office supply inventory
   C. Land
   D. Prepaid expenses

2. Which of the following cannot be calculated as depreciating in value?
   A. Furniture
   B. Supplies
   C. Equipment
   D. Land

3. Dr. Silverton owns a family medical practice. The practice prepays for a maintenance contract on office equipment at the rate of $600 for 6 months. The most recent contract period started December 1 and will cover the months of December through May. The financial records of the practice are maintained on a calendar-year basis. How much of the maintenance contract will be booked as a prepaid expense as of December 31?

4. Dr. Silverton's practice is in a community with a relatively high percentage of low-income households. At the end of the fiscal year, the accounts receivable for the practice totals $60,000. Half of that amount is from insurance claims not yet paid and are assumed to be fully collectible. The other half is made up of receivables from private-pay patients. Dr. Silverton treats a few families knowing that they are unable to pay the full amount charged and has estimated that the uncollectible portion of receivables from private pay patients is 20 percent. What is the allowance for uncollectible accounts receivable?

5. Using the definition of capital assets established in Medicare regulations, which of the following would be treated as non-current assets under furniture and equipment?
   A. Cellular phones costing $400
   B. Lakeview Medical's initial stock of disposable medical supplies costing $1,200

continued

C. An examination table costing $2,000

D. Office furniture costing $4,500

E. All of the above

6. Define the terms **depreciation** and **accumulated depreciation**.

_____

_____

_____

7. Tacey's Pharmacy offers free prescription delivery to customers. The pharmacy maintains its financial records on a calendar-year basis. At the end of June, Tacey's purchases a new delivery vehicle costing $20,000. They plan to use the vehicle in the business for 5 years and expect the vehicle will have a trade-in value after 5 years of $5,000. What is the annual charge for depreciation on this asset? What would be the net value in the first year of purchase?

8. A large urban health maintenance organization (HMO) purchases a vacant office building to house expanded administrative functions for $300,000. Prior to using the building, renovations costing $100,000 are completed. The renovated building has an estimated useful life of 27.5 years, with no residual value. What is the annual charge for depreciation?

9. Plastic Surgery Associates buys surgical lights for $10,000. The lights have an estimated salvage value of $2,000 and a useful life of 5 years. Calculate the straight-line depreciation.

10. Dr. Kahn is projecting his total assets for the year 2021. He is tallying the 2019 and 2020 current and non-current assets to determine the range of total assets for 2021. Calculate the total current, total non-current, and total assets for each year.

Assets	2019	2020
Current Assets		
Cash	$ 24,000.00	$ 10,000.00
Account Receivables	$ 35,000.00	$ 44,000.00
Inventory	$ 68,000.00	$ 60,000.00
Prepaid Expenses	$ 3,000.00	$ 2,000.00
Total Current Assets	a.	b.
Non-Current Assets		
Equipment	$ 100,000.00	$ 80,000.00
Office Furniture	$ 20,000.00	$ 15,000.00
Handheld computers	$ 15,000.00	$ 20,000.00
Total Non-Current Assets	c.	d.
Total Assets	e.	f.

Liabilities

Liabilities are all the debts of the business as of the date of the balance sheet. **Current liabilities**, such as recurring monthly bills for supplies and utilities, are those debts that will be paid within the next 12 months. Debts that will be paid in a period longer than 1 year are categorized as **non-current liabilities**.

Current Liabilities

Liabilities, like assets, are divided into current and non-current on the balance sheet. Current liabilities will include all debts of the business that will be paid during the upcoming 12 months. Current liabilities include:

- Accounts payable
- Accrued liabilities
- Portion of long-term debt that will be paid during the next year.
- Other current liabilities

Figure 6-7 shows an example of a current liabilities section of the balance sheet.

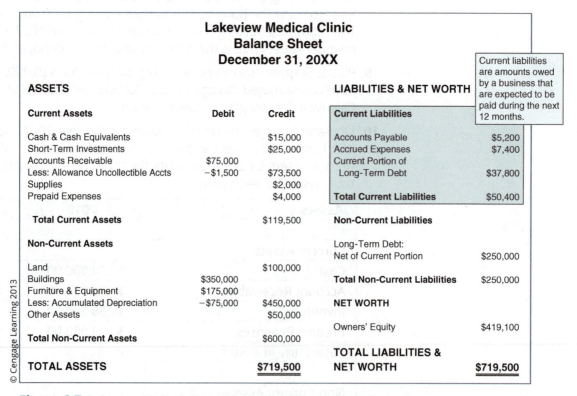

Lakeview Medical Clinic
Balance Sheet
December 31, 20XX

Current liabilities are amounts owed by a business that are expected to be paid during the next 12 months.

ASSETS				LIABILITIES & NET WORTH	
Current Assets	**Debit**	**Credit**		**Current Liabilities**	
Cash & Cash Equivalents		$15,000		Accounts Payable	$5,200
Short-Term Investments		$25,000		Accrued Expenses	$7,400
Accounts Receivable	$75,000			Current Portion of	
Less: Allowance Uncollectible Accts	−$1,500	$73,500		Long-Term Debt	$37,800
Supplies		$2,000			
Prepaid Expenses		$4,000		**Total Current Liabilities**	$50,400
Total Current Assets		$119,500		**Non-Current Liabilities**	
Non-Current Assets				Long-Term Debt:	
				Net of Current Portion	$250,000
Land		$100,000			
Buildings	$350,000			**Total Non-Current Liabilities**	$250,000
Furniture & Equipment	$175,000				
Less: Accumulated Depreciation	−$75,000	$450,000		**NET WORTH**	
Other Assets		$50,000			
				Owners' Equity	$419,100
Total Non-Current Assets		$600,000			
				TOTAL LIABILITIES &	
TOTAL ASSETS		$719,500		**NET WORTH**	$719,500

© Cengage Learning 2013

Figure 6-7 Lakeview Medical Clinic Current Liabilities on the Balance Sheet

Accounts Payable

Accounts payable are payments due for goods delivered or services used near the end of the fiscal year where the vendor has not been paid by the date of the financial statement. In January, a medical practice pays the office bills, including the utility bills for December and medical supplies that were ordered and delivered during December. The total of these unpaid bills for December goods and services will be included on the balance sheet as accounts payables at the end of the year.

Accrued Expenses

Accrued expenses are used to account for bills paid early in the new fiscal year where the total amount of the expense needs to be split between the old and new fiscal year. Commonly used items for accrued expenses are accrued payroll and accrued interest payable.

Example 6-3

To illustrate the concept of accrued expenses: A hospital employee is paid $500 per week for a 40-hour work week and is paid every 2 weeks. The employee's first paycheck in January in the amount of $1,000 before taxes and deductions is for one week worked in December and a week worked in January. The $500 wages for the week worked in December will show on the financial statements of the hospital as an accrued liability. Payroll costs for December, even though paid in January, are costs of generating December revenues and need to be posted to that accounting period.

A second accrued expense is accrued interest on outstanding debt. Lakeview Medical Clinic has an outstanding bank loan for the purchase of a major piece of medical equipment. Payments of principal and interest are made quarterly on January 31, April 30, July 31, and October 31. The interest payment made on January 31 includes interest charges for the months of November, December, and January. The balance sheet for December 31 will show accrued interest payable equal to two-thirds of the interest payment (for the months of November and December) to be made on January 31. The January 31 payment to the bank included a principal payment and $1,500 of interest on the loan. $1,000 in interest is an expense for the prior fiscal year and is posted as an accrued liability on the December 31 financial statements. The $500 interest paid for January will be an expense for the new fiscal year.

Current Portion of Long-Term Debt

Current portion of long-term debt is the amount of principal on outstanding loans that is scheduled to be paid during the 12 months of the current fiscal year. The equipment loan for Lakeview Medical is in the second year of repayment on an original 5-year loan and calls for a payment of both principal and interest on each quarterly payment date. The medical facility building is subject to a mortgage with a remaining life of 12 years. The current portion of the two loans combined is $37,800, representing the amount of principal that will be paid in the current fiscal year.

Other Current Liabilities

Other current liabilities will include any liabilities of the business that are not accounted for in other liability categories. The most common use of the category of other current liabilities in medical practice is **deferred revenues** in HMOs. Some HMO medical facilities receive their revenues based on capitation rates, the monthly amount paid for each covered individual. In the final month of a fiscal year, an HMO facility receives payment to provide care to patients for the first month of the new fiscal year. This payment represents an obligation to provide care in the future and is a liability to the facility since costs related to this payment will be incurred in the new fiscal year. The payment is recorded as a deferred revenue and will appear as a liability on the year-end financial records of the HMO facility. In the balance sheet example in Figure 6-7, Lakeview Medical does not have any year-end liabilities that would be categorized as other current liabilities.

Non-Current Liabilities

Non-current liabilities are amounts owed by a business that are expected to be paid on a future date more than 12 months away, as shown in Figure 6-8. The most common example of a non-current liability is the balance on an outstanding loan that will not be paid during the current fiscal year.

Long-term debt: net of current portion is the amount of principal on outstanding debt that is scheduled to be paid in future fiscal years. Again, using the Lakeview Medical example, the balance sheet at Figure 6-1 shows the total balance due on the equipment loan and the mortgage is $287,800, with $37,800 due to be repaid during the current fiscal year. The balance of $250,000 will be repaid in future fiscal years and will be shown as long-term debt net of current portion. Details on the loans will be included in the notes to the financial statements.

Lakeview Medical Clinic
Balance Sheet
December 31, 20XX

ASSETS			LIABILITIES & NET WORTH	
Current Assets	Debit	Credit	**Current Liabilities**	
Cash & Cash Equivalents		$15,000	Accounts Payable	$5,200
Short-Term Investments		$25,000	Accrued Expenses	$7,400
Accounts Receivable	$75,000		Current Portion of	
Less: Allowance Uncollectible Accts	−$1,500	$73,500	Long-Term Debt	$37,800
Supplies		$2,000		
Prepaid Expenses		$4,000	**Total Current Liabilities**	$50,400
Total Current Assets		$119,500	**Non-Current Liabilities**	
Non-Current Assets			Long-Term Debt:	
			Net of Current Portion	$250,000
Land		$100,000		
Buildings	$350,000		**Total Non-Current Liabilities**	$250,000
Furniture & Equipment	$175,000			
Less: Accumulated Depreciation	−$75,000	$450,000	**NET WORTH**	
Other Assets		$50,000		
			Owners' Equity	$419,100
Total Non-Current Assets		$600,000		
			TOTAL LIABILITIES &	
TOTAL ASSETS		**$719,500**	**NET WORTH**	**$719,500**

> Non-current liabilities are amounts owed by a business that are expected to be paid at a date in the future more than 12 months away.

© Cengage Learning 2013

Figure 6-8 Lakeview Medical Clinic Non-Current Liabilities on the Balance Sheet

Comprehension Check 6.3

In the following list, identify which are current or long-term liabilities:

Long-term loan

Income tax

Deferred tax liabilities

Payable notes

Interest payable

Bonds payable

Notes payable

Net Worth

The net worth of any business is the difference between total assets and total liabilities as shown in Figure 6-9.

Referring to Figure 6-6, the net worth would be determined by using the net worth equation: $719,500 (total assets of the clinic) − $50,400 (total clinic current liabilities) − $260,000 (total clinic non-current liabilities) = $419,100. The net worth of the clinic is $419,100.

The terminology used in the net worth section of the balance sheet depends on the legal structure of the business.

- **Owners' equity** is used in sole proprietorships and partnerships to show the ownership right of the proprietor or partners in the business.

- **Capital stock** and **retained earnings** are the standard terms used for a corporation. Capital stock is the funds invested by the stockholders and retained earnings are the accumulated excess of revenues over expenses generated by the business. Capital stock and retained earnings combine to show the **stockholders' equity** in the corporation.

- **Net assets** is the accounting term that represents the ownership by the community in a facility that is owned by a local government.

- **Fund balance** is the term used by not-for-profit organizations.

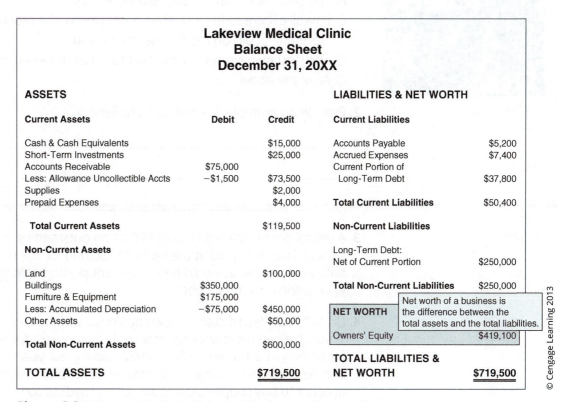

Lakeview Medical Clinic
Balance Sheet
December 31, 20XX

ASSETS			LIABILITIES & NET WORTH	
Current Assets	Debit	Credit	**Current Liabilities**	
Cash & Cash Equivalents		$15,000	Accounts Payable	$5,200
Short-Term Investments		$25,000	Accrued Expenses	$7,400
Accounts Receivable	$75,000		Current Portion of	
Less: Allowance Uncollectible Accts	−$1,500	$73,500	Long-Term Debt	$37,800
Supplies		$2,000		
Prepaid Expenses		$4,000	**Total Current Liabilities**	$50,400
Total Current Assets		$119,500	**Non-Current Liabilities**	
Non-Current Assets			Long-Term Debt:	
			Net of Current Portion	$250,000
Land		$100,000		
Buildings	$350,000		**Total Non-Current Liabilities**	$250,000
Furniture & Equipment	$175,000			
Less: Accumulated Depreciation	−$75,000	$450,000	**NET WORTH**	
Other Assets		$50,000	Owners' Equity	$419,100
Total Non-Current Assets		$600,000	**TOTAL LIABILITIES &**	
TOTAL ASSETS		$719,500	**NET WORTH**	$719,500

Net worth of a business is the difference between the total assets and the total liabilities.

Figure 6-9 Lakeview Medical Clinic Net Worth on the Balance Sheet

Comprehension Check 6.4

1. Gadar Abbas, RN, decided to create a nonprofit agency for single-parent families to help them find community resources. What type of legal structure would her business have?

2. Dr. Iban decided to open up his own medical practice where he owns the business solely. What type of legal structure would his business have?

3. Medical For Us is a government agency that specializes in providing medical services for the disadvantaged youth. What type of legal structure would this be?

4. Sage Zin is part of a corporation of dental organizations. The stockholders invest in capital stock. What type of legal structure would their business have?

Knowledge Check

6.2

1. Which of the following would be shown as current liabilities for a medical practice maintaining financial records on a calendar-year basis?
   A. The December electric bill, paid in January
   B. Payroll expenses for days that employees of the practice worked in December, paid on the first payroll in January
   C. The January payment for medical supplies delivered in December
   D. All of the above

2. Provide an example of a non-current liability.

   _____

   _____

   _____

3. A dental organization has $725,000 as an outstanding loan, for which the principal must be paid at the rate of $150,000 for the next 5 years. In the balance sheet, what would be the current portion of long-term debt and what is the remaining debt?

4. Dr. Mills decided to start his own business, which he entitled Express Vision. He had been working as an ophthalmologist for Vision World for many years, but he decided 2022 was a great year to start his own business. To start his own business, he needed to take out cash from his account to buy supplies, computers, and medical software. In addition, he hired several employees, so he had to obtain a long-term bank loan to pay salaries and allow for taxes for his business. The following list shows Dr. Mills' assets and liabilities.

continued

Express Vision	
Balance Sheet	
Saturday, January 22, 2022	
Short-Term Assets	
Cash	$10,000
Supplies	$76,000
Total Short-Term Assets	
Long-Term Assets	
Computers	$25,000
Medical Software	$28,000
Total Long-Term Assets	
Liabilities and Owner's Equity	
Bank Loan	$100,000
Salaries Payable	$12,000
Taxes	$5,000
TOTAL LIABILITIES	
TOTAL LIABILITIES AND OWNER'S EQUITY	

Key Chapter Equation: Accounting

The Accounting Equation can be written in various ways, such as:
Owner's Equity = Assets − Liabilities
Assets = Liabilities + Owner's Equity

A. Calculate Dr. Mills' total short-term assets.
B. Calculate Dr. Mills' long-term assets.
C. Calculate Dr. Mills' liabilities.
D. Calculate Dr. Mills' ownership equity.

5. The reader of the financial statements of a medical facility sees the heading Stockholders' Equity in the net worth section of the balance sheet. This indicates that the legal structure of the facility is a:
A. Partnership
B. Corporation
C. Sole proprietorship
D. Facility owned by a local government
E. Not-for-profit

6. Dr. Tran owns an urgent clinic. Her total assets are $900,000. Using the following information, determine Dr. Tran's current liabilities, non-current liabilities, and net worth:

Liabilities and Net Worth	
Current Liabilities	
Accounts Payable	$ 4,500.00
Long-Term Debt	$ 45,000.00
Deferred Revenues	$ 7,000.00
Total Current Liabilities	a.
Non-Current Liabilities	
Long-Term Debt	$ 60,000.00
Total Non-Current Liabilities	b.
Net Worth: Owner's Equity	c.
Total Liabilities & Net Worth	d.

7. Which of the following are assets and which are liabilities?
Accounts payable
Accrued expenses
Supplies
Long term debt
Prepaid expenses
Cash

8. Dr. Jay is opening an emergency vet service within his community in January. He invested $425,000 cash into the business. Dr. Jay bought vet supplies, equipment, vet software, and office equipment for $200,000. In addition, there is a long-term loan for $50,000. What is his total owner's equity?

Key Concepts

- The balance sheet of any business represents the book value of its financial position at a fixed point in time.

- The assets of the business are all the items of measurable financial value owned by the business. Assets are divided between current assets, items of value expected to be used within 12 months, and non-current assets, those having a useful life of longer than 1 year.

- Depreciation is used to measure the loss in value of capital assets as these assets reduce in value over time from either wearing out or obsolescence. Accumulated depreciation is the total of the annual charges for depreciation for each individual asset since that asset was placed in use.

- Liabilities on the balance sheet are debts owed by the business as of the date of the balance sheet. As with assets, liabilities are divided between current and non-current. Current liabilities will be paid within 12 months, and non-current liabilities will be paid at a point in time longer than 1 year away.

- The net worth of any business is the difference between total assets and total liabilities.

The Income Statement

Chapter Objectives

After completing this chapter, readers should be able to:

- Describe the accounting treatment of revenues and the concept of net medical services revenue.

- Classify payroll and other expenses on the income statement.

- Discuss government requirements for minimum pay and overtime pay.

- Explain the concept of net income.

- Demonstrate an understanding of income statement analysis.

Chapter Glossary

Balance billing is the prohibited practice of billing patients for amounts greater than contract rates for medical services.

Current ratio compares the balance sheet value of current assets to current liabilities.

Debt-to-net-worth ratio compares the debt (liabilities owed) of the business to net worth.

Fair Labor Standards Act (FLSA) of 1938 establishes minimum wage rates and regulates the requirement for overtime pay.

Gross medical service revenues are what the medical facility would have received if all services provided were billed and paid at the full price charged to private-pay patients.

Gross pay is the amount of the employee's periodic paycheck before taxes and other deductions.

The **income statement** reports revenues, expenses, and net income over the period of time covered in the report.

Net income is the excess of revenues over expenses for the period of time accounted for in the income statement.

Net medical service revenue is the amount of revenue expected to be received by the medical facility for services provided.

Net pay is the actual amount of the employee's periodic paycheck.

Quick ratio is the current assets of cash, short-term investments, and accounts receivable compared to current liabilities.

Introduction

The balance sheet describes the financial position of a medical facility at a certain point in time, in this case the last day of the fiscal year. There are various ratios that can be used to determine the financial longevity of a medical facility. When determining the financial aspect of an organization, the balance sheet and the income statement ratio can be used.

The balance sheet is utilized to determine the short-term financial status of an organization. The two ratios used are the **current ratio** and **quick ratio**.

The current ratio compares the balance sheet value of current assets to current liabilities. A ratio under 1.00 indicates that the company's debts due in a year or less are greater than its assets—cash or other short-term assets expected to be converted to cash within a year or less. A current ratio of less than 1.00 may seem alarming, although different situations can negatively affect the current ratio in a solid company.

In theory, the higher the current ratio, the more capable a company is of paying its obligations because it has a larger proportion of short-term asset value relative to the value of its short-term liabilities. However, although a high ratio—say, more than 3.00—could indicate that the company can cover its current liabilities three times, it also may indicate that it is not using its current assets efficiently.

Key Chapter Equation: Current Ratio

The current ratio equation is:
Current Ratio = Current Assets/Current Liabilities

In addition, the quick ratio is a second comparison to indicate the facility's ability to meet current obligations. In the quick ratio, only the current assets of cash, short-term investments, and accounts receivable are compared to current liabilities. Short-term investments and accounts receivable are compared to current liabilities.

The quick ratio looks at only the most liquid assets that a company has available to service short-term debts and obligations. Liquid assets are those that can be quickly and easily converted into cash to pay those bills. A quick ratio 1.0 or higher indicates the business is healthy.

> **Key Chapter Equation: Quick Ratio**
>
> The quick ratio equation is:
> **Quick Ratio Equation = Cash + Short-Term Investments + Net Accounts Receivable/Current Liabilities**

Comprehension Check 7.1

Using the following data on current assets and liabilities, calculate the current ratio and the quick ratio for the medical facility.

Current Assets	Debit	Credit	Current Liabilities	
Cash & Cash Equivalent		$8,000	Accounts Payable	$5,000
Short-Term Investments		$60,000	Accrued Expenses	$7,500
Accounts Receivable	$25,000		Current Portion	
Less: Uncollectable	$5,000		Long-Term Debt	$10,000
Supplies		$2,000		
Prepaid Expenses		$5,000		
Total Current Assets		$75,000	Total Current Liabilities	$22,500

Comprehension Check 7.2

Using the following data, calculate the medical facilities' current ratios. Based on the current ratios, which of the following medical facilities is the healthiest financially?

In Millions	Delphy Medical Facility	Johnson Medical Facility	Aztric Medical Facility
Current Assets	$18,000	$29,000	$18,000
Current Liabilities	$24,000	$30,000	$28,000
Quick Ratio			

A ratio that compares the debt (liabilities owed) of the business to net worth is the **debt-to-net-worth ratio**. A ratio of 1.0 shows the business with debt is equal to the net worth. A ratio of less than 1.0 shows the net worth is greater than total debt. This ratio indicates the ability of a business to meet obligations for payment on long-term debt.

Key Chapter Equation: Debt-to-Net-Worth Ratio

The debt-to-net-worth ratio is:

Net Worth = Total Assets − Total Liabilities
Debt-to-Net-Worth Equation
Debt-to-Net-Worth Ratio = Total Liabilities/Net Worth

Comprehension Check 7.3

Using the following data, determine the debt-to-net-worth ratio for each urgent care facility.

Urgent Care	Liabilities	Net Worth
Hanja Urgent Care	$5,000,000	$7,000,000
Zahani Urgent Care	$4,000,000	$5,000,000

The companion accounting report to the balance sheet is the **income statement**, shown in Figure 7-1. The income statement reports on revenues, expenses, and net income over the period of time covered in the report. In comparison, the balance sheet shows balances of what is owned and what is owed at a certain point in time. The income statement presents revenues and expenses over a period of time. The income statement will always be prepared annually. It can also be prepared on a more frequent basis, monthly or quarterly, to meet the financial information needs of management and other interested parties.

Revenues

Net medical service revenues reflects the revenues expected to be received by the medical facility for services provided. **Gross medical service revenues** are what the facility would have received if all services provided were billed and paid at the full price charged to private-pay patients. Almost all medical facilities have contracts in place with a variety of group health insurance providers and accept payments from government programs such as Medicare and Medicaid. The total of the deductibles, patient copayments, and government or insurance reimbursements makes up the revenues to the medical facility for services provided to patients covered by these plans. Each individual insurance program and government

Lakeview Medical Clinic
Income Statement
For the Year Ending December 31, 20XX

REVENUES:

Gross medical services revenue	$1,250,000	
Less: Contractual adjustments	−250,000	
Net medical services revenue		$1,000,000
Other income		5,000
Total Revenues		**1,005,000**

EXPENSES:

Salaries and benefits	750,000
Supplies	25,000
Contract services	15,000
Bad debt expense	1,500
Insurance	40,000
Depreciation & Amortization	22,000
Interest expense	20,000
Other expense	5,000
Total Expenses	**878,500**

INCOME:

Net Income	**$126,500**

Figure 7-1 Lakeview Medical Clinic Income Statement

programs such as Medicare have their own deductibles and copayment requirements; the medical facility is responsible for monitoring the plans to ensure that the patient pays the proper amount.

Contractual Reimbursement

The reimbursement rates from these contracts will be less than the pricing schedule of the facility for private-pay patients. Hospitals, as a requirement of their certificate of need, are required to provide charity care to indigent members of their local community. As noted previously, the business of providing medical services is unique in that medical facilities may not know how much they will be paid until the bill is actually paid by a third party, either an insurance company or the government. Modern computer technology has removed a large amount of this uncertainty, allowing the facility to use a database of current contract rates to accurately determine the book amounts expected to be received from insurance providers and government programs.

Example 7-1

Mr. Timkins is referred by his family physician to Digestive Health Associates for a routine screening colonoscopy. Mr. Timkins is covered by Blue Cross/Blue Shield, a group health insurer through his employer. He has met his annual deductible for the year and has no copayment requirement for this procedure. On September 14, the date of the colonoscopy, Digestive Health will make the following entry into their accounting records, showing the medical service performed at their standard billing rate, as shown in Figure 7-2.

ACCOUNTING ENTRY

ACCOUNT NUMBER	DESCRIPTION	DEBIT	CREDIT
	Accounts Receivable	1,120.00	
	Medical Services Revenue		1,120.00

© Cengage Learning 2013

Figure 7-2 Service Account Entry by Digestive Health

Later that week, Digestive Health fills out the request for insurance reimbursement with Blue Cross/Blue Shield and submits the request for payment. Based on the rates in the current contract with the insurance provider, Digestive Health receives $340.00 for the colonoscopy. At the time funds are received, Digestive Health makes the following accounting entry (see Figure 7-3) to record the receipt of cash, adjust medical services revenues to the contract rate, and close the accounts receivable for this procedure.

ACCOUNTING ENTRY

ACCOUNT NUMBER	DESCRIPTION	DEBIT	CREDIT
	Cash	340.00	
	Medical Services Revenue	780.00	
	Accounts Receivable		1,120.00

© Cengage Learning 2013

Figure 7-3 Payment Received Account Entry by Digestive Health

In this example, revenues are adjusted to the contractual rates for payment. The use of this accounting treatment balances the revenue account to the contractual amounts paid for medical services. It is also a common practice to maintain the revenue account at the full rates charged by the facility for its private-pay patients. The medical facility will then use an account titled **contractual adjustments** to accumulate payments for medical service received at the lower contract rates. At the end of the accounting period, this account will show the medical facility the financial impact of accepting the lower contractual amounts as compared to the facility's full rates. Either accounting treatment is acceptable.

Balance Billing

Balance billing is a practice prohibited under all group insurance contracts and government programs. Medical facilities are required to accept the combination of **copayment** and deductible contributions from the patient, and insurance reimbursements at contract rates, as full payment for the medical services provided. The facility must adjust any medical services revenue and accounts receivable that remain after the proper payments have been received from both the patient and the insurance provider. **The patient may not be billed for any amount above the contractual rate**. The combination of the two accounting entries in Figures 7-2 and 7-3 posts the proper amount to net medical services revenue. The full service charge of $1,120 is posted as revenue in Figure 7-2 and is then reduced by $780 in Figure 7-3 to arrive at the proper revenue for the procedure of $340. The alternative treatment is to post the $780 adjustment to revenue to the contractual adjustments account discussed previously. In either case, the net result is revenues received of $340, not the $1,120 originally posted for the procedure.

Other income will include any revenues received by the medical facility that are not related to providing medical services to patients. This category would include any lease revenue, interest earned on bank and money market accounts, and any salvage value received from the sale of equipment replaced in the normal course of business. In the event that any other income items are material to the financial operations of the facility, they would be listed separately as income items.

Knowledge Check 7.1

1. How can ratios be used in determining the financial condition of a medical facility?

2. The year-end balance sheet of a hospital shows total liabilities of $5,500,000, including a bank note to expand the facility. Net worth of the hospital is $3,000,000. What is the debt-to-net-worth ratio?

3. Explain the difference between gross medical services revenue and net medical services revenue.

_____

_____

_____

4. What is balance billing, and why is it a prohibited practice?

_____

_____

_____

continued

5. Mrs. Foster meets with her family physician complaining of flu-like symptoms that have continued for almost a week. She has group health insurance through her employer, with the contract requiring a $30.00 office visit copayment from the patient. The facility's standard billing rate for a routine office visit is $150.00. Complete the following journal entry to record the cash received from Mrs. Foster, the amount due from the insurance company, and the medical services revenue:

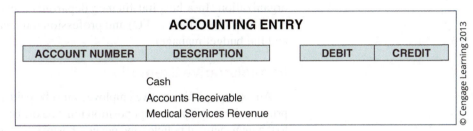

6. Based on the facts in question 5, Mrs. Foster's insurance company pays the contract rate of $55.00 for the medical service. This is in addition to the patient's required copayment. Complete the following journal entry to record cash received, adjust medical services revenue, and clear the accounts receivable:

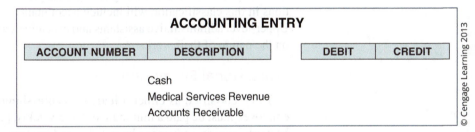

Expenses: Salaries and Benefits

For medical organizations, the largest single area of expense is the salaries and benefits paid to employees. To attract and retain employees, these facilities need to have competitive pay and benefits packages. Base levels of pay and compensation for overtime work are governed by the **Fair Labor Standards Act (FLSA) of 1938**. The current federal minimum wage is $7.25 per hour, established by Congress effective July 24, 2009. A number of states have implemented minimum wage laws that provide for a minimum wage higher than the federal requirement. All businesses need to monitor any changes in either the federal or state minimum wage laws.

Exempt and Nonexempt Employees

FLSA also established the concept of **exempt** and **nonexempt** employees to clarify which of the employees in the organization are eligible for overtime pay. In general, overtime at the rate of one and one-half (1.5) times the employee's hourly rate of pay needs to be paid to nonexempt employees working more than forty (40) hours in a standard workweek. Overtime is not paid to exempt employees. The law provides for six classes of employees exempt from the requirement to pay overtime.

Executive Exemption

To qualify as an executive exempt from overtime pay, the employee must be paid a minimum of $455 weekly, be actively involved in the management of the organization, supervise at least two full-time employees, and be involved in the hiring and firing process. The employee must not spend more than 20 percent of the workweek involved in activities that are nonexempt under the law. In medical facilities, employees exempt under this classification will include the top management team of the organization. In a hospital finance department, exempt employees will include the chief financial officer (CFO) and professional managers such as the chief accountant and the budget manager.

Administrative Exemption

An exempt administrative employee must be paid a minimum of $455 weekly, and the primary duties of the exempt position must be office and nonmanual work that is related to the management policies and general business of the organization and that requires the use of discretion and independent judgment. A hospital's risk manager will be an exempt administrative employee. The risk manager may not have a staff to supervise but works only under general supervision and will independently make decisions and judgments affecting the entire organization.

Exempt positions will commonly require specialized training and experience and may include special assignments assigned by management. In medical facilities, exempt positions in this classification will include accountants and human resources professionals. Upper-level administrative assistants and executive secretaries may also be exempt based on the nature of their work.

Professional Exemption

To be classified as either a **learned professional** or a **creative professional**, the employee must be paid a minimum of $455 weekly, primary duties for the position must be work requiring advanced knowledge and training, and duties must include work that requires the use of discretion and judgment. Positions exempt under this classification will generally require licenses to practice, such as physicians, physician assistants, psychologists, and lawyers. Teachers are considered to be exempt professionals, while nurses are generally nonexempt. The distinctions between exempt and nonexempt professionals have evolved from legal actions concerning overtime pay.

Computer Employee Exemption

An exempt employee in the field of information technology must be paid a minimum of $455 weekly and be employed in a skilled position such as programmer, systems analyst, or software engineer. Primary duties of the employee must be in the field of systems analysis and the development, design, documentation, and modification of computerized systems.

Outside Sales Exemption

Primary duties of the employee exempt from overtime related to outside sales must be in making sales away from the employer's place of business. Sales are defined in the regulation to include soliciting and obtaining contracts for goods, services, or the use of property.

Highly Compensated Employees Exemption

Employees earning $100,000 or more per year and performing at least one of the duties listed for exempt executive, administrative, or professional positions are also exempt from the overtime requirement.

In a smaller medical office, the physician and the practice manager are exempt from the overtime requirements, while the rest of the employees will be eligible for overtime pay. In larger medical facilities, such as hospitals, the human resources department will be responsible for reviewing each of the positions within the organization to determine the exempt or nonexempt status of each employee based on the nature of their work and the exemptions available under FLSA.

Comprehension Check 7.4

1. Dr. Zinn is employed at Saunders Medical Practice. Dr. Zinn is involved in teaching surgical technicians surgical skills so they are prepared to enter the workplace. Dr. Zinn has to maintain a professional license along with a surgical certificate to meet the medical facility's educational requirement. This is an example of which type of exemption?

2. Owen Bowers is employed at Zeller Rehabilitation Center. The position requires human resource responsibilities along with assisting the risk manager at the hospital. Owen has specialized training in both areas and enjoys the ability to assist the two departments based on the center's needs. This is an example of which type of exemption?

3. Amelia Benn was just promoted to Director of Operations at Zynsky Dental Organization. The organization has more than 500 employees. Amelia has three direct employees that report to her. Her position consists of actively being involved in the hiring process to ensure that the dental organization is operating efficiently. This is an example of which type of exemption?

Common Payroll Periods

The days of the weekly pay envelope, with employees receiving cash for the week's work on Friday afternoon, are long gone. Employers pay their employees by check or with direct deposit of the employee's paycheck into their bank account to avoid issues of lost checks or fraudulent changes made to checks. Most businesses pay their employees on either a biweekly basis (26 payrolls per year) or a semimonthly basis (24 payrolls per year, generally paid on the 15th and last working day of the month). Exempt employees will have a stated annual salary and be paid in either 26 or 24 equal installments. Hourly employees will have an established hourly rate of pay and be paid based on the number of hours worked during the pay period. The physician who owns a medical practice or the partners involved in a medical facility will receive payments for services each payroll period called **draws**. Draws are treated as a business expense assuming that they are reported to the Internal Revenue Service as salaries paid.

Taxes

There is a major difference between the salary of the position or the number of hours worked at the hourly rate of pay (**gross pay**) and the actual amount of the paycheck (**net pay**). When a new employee is hired, one of the first items of paperwork to be completed is the federal W-4 form **Employee's Withholding Allowance Certificate**. This form lists the marital status of the employee, the number of dependents claimed for federal income tax purposes, and the number of additional exemptions based on itemized deductions that exceed the standard deduction. Employees also have the option to have additional taxes withheld, based on individual circumstances. This form tells the payroll clerk how much of each paycheck needs to be withheld from the employee's pay and remitted to the federal government for income taxes.

Employees have the ability to reduce the amount of their gross pay subject to federal income tax. Many employers have established pretax retirement plans, where employee payroll contributions to retirement savings accounts are deposited on a pretax basis. Also, employee healthcare insurance plans can be structured where the employee share of insurance premiums and deposits to a healthcare savings account (HSA) are on a pretax basis. When authorized by the employee, these amounts are withheld from the employee's pay and deposited with the appropriate retirement and healthcare provider.

With very few exceptions, all employees are subject to both Social Security and Medicare taxes. Social Security is taxed at the rate of 6.2 percent of pay (4.2 percent as a 2-year reduction for 2011 and 2012 to stimulate the economy) subject to a maximum amount established annually. For 2012, the maximum was $110,100. Earnings above that level are not subject to Social Security tax. Medicare is taxed at the rate of 1.45 percent and does not have a maximum income subject to the tax. For each employee, the employer is required to match both the Social Security and Medicare taxes. These taxes paid by the employer show as an expense in the financial records of the medical facility.

At the end of each year, each employee will receive a federal W-2 form **Wage and Tax Statement**. This form will detail the gross pay earned by the employee, adjustments to gross pay to determine federally taxable income, and the amounts of income tax, Social Security, and Medicare withheld.

Benefits

The financial records of most medical facilities will also show costs related to employee benefits. Benefits that are standard to many medical facilities will include the employer contribution to employee health insurance, employer contribution to a retirement plan, and perhaps employer-paid life or dental insurance.

Take, for example, the following scenario in Example 7-2 of how benefits impact the expenses of a healthcare facility.

Example 7-2

High Plains Life Care Facility provides a retirement savings plan for employees where the medical facility agrees to match employee contributions to the plan up to a maximum of 5 percent of each employee's pay. Participation in the plan is voluntary. The cost to High Plains to match employee contributions is shown on the financial records as an employee benefit cost. The facility also has a healthcare insurance plan benefit for employees. The insurance plan ensures that the facility will pay the cost of the monthly premium of a single employee at a current cost of $400 monthly. The employee has the opportunity to purchase healthcare insurance for other family members at group insurance rates. The $400 monthly contributed by High Plains will be shown as facility expenses under employee benefits.

Other Expenses

As noted, salaries and benefits will comprise the majority of the annual expenses of a medical facility. However, the costs of doing business will also include a number of other expense areas, which follow.

Supplies

These include the expenses of purchasing all of the routine disposable items used in the business. For medical facilities, this will include both office supplies and medical supplies. Many income statements for medical facilities will show both supply expense categories separately. This area of expense will also include items that have a useful life of longer than 1 year that do not meet the minimum cost level to be included in capital assets.

Contract Services

Contract services include the expenses for all of the services needed to operate the business. This category would likely include janitorial and after-hours paging services. Medical facilities may choose to have staff employees provide these types of services. In those cases, the costs will be included under salaries and benefits.

Bad Debt Expense

Bad debt expense is the estimate of the amount of accounts receivable on the balance sheet that will not be paid. This expense category will not include the costs of charity care or amounts paid under contractual relationships that are less than the facility's normal billing rates. Those amounts have already been adjusted in calculating net medical services revenues.

Insurance

Insurance is the cost of transferring risk to others. Businesses will carry a range of insurance coverage to protect against financial loss. Homeowners will transfer the cost of rebuilding their homes after a fire to an insurance company with the purchase of homeowner's insurance and the payment of annual premiums. Medical facilities use insurance companies in a similar fashion, purchasing insurance against business risks such as fire, premises liability, and medical malpractice. The subject of managing financial risk is covered in Chapter 12.

Depreciation and Amortization

Depreciation and amortization are the annual charges that represent the loss in value as assets are used up in the operations of the business. Depreciation and amortization were discussed in Chapter 6.

Interest and Other Expenses

Interest expense is the annual cost of the time value of money. Amounts paid out to reduce the amount of the loan show as a reduction of the principal balance on the loan and will not appear on the income statement, while annual amounts paid as interest are shown as an expense.

Other expense, like other revenue, is a category used to account for any expenses that do not fit into any other expense category.

Net Income

Net income is the excess of revenues over expenses for the period of time accounted for in the income statement. In the business world, this item is commonly referred to as "profit" or "the bottom line." The terminology used in not-for-profit organizations is **change in net assets**. Any business, either through mismanagement or economic conditions, can suffer losses. In these cases, net income will be a negative number showing that expenses exceeded revenues for the period.

Knowledge Check

7.2

1. Philip Tryon is the CFO for Northport Regional Hospital. In his position, he supervises a staff of eight and participates in making key financial decisions for the hospital. Is Mr. Tryon an exempt or a nonexempt employee for overtime under FLSA? Why?

_____

_____

_____

2. Rebecca Thompson is the maintenance supervisor for Northport Regional Hospital. She supervises a staff of four but spends approximately 50 percent of her time performing hands-on maintenance functions for the hospital. Is Ms. Thompson an exempt or a nonexempt employee for overtime under FLSA? Why?

_____

_____

_____

3. A home healthcare agency has a physician as the executive director and six employees providing direct care services to patients. The accounting records of the agency show the following items:

Salaries and overtime pay	$425,000
Social Security/Medicare paid by agency	$30,000
Social Security/Medicare paid by employees	$30,000
Employer deposits—retirement savings	$15,000
Employer contribution—health insurance	$42,000

Calculate the total payroll expenses for this agency.

_____

_____

_____

4. Which of the following items will appear on the income statement of a medical facility?
   A. The cost of accounts receivable written off as bad debts
   B. Supplies purchased for the facility during the year
   C. Payroll and benefit costs paid by the facility
   D. Depreciation of capital assets
   E. All of the above

continued

5. Dr. Foster's primary care practice had net medical service revenue of $500,000 for the year. Salaries and benefits for the year, including draws for Dr. Foster, were $350,000. Other operating expenses, excluding payments on a bank loan, were $100,000. Payments on the bank loan for the year were $50,000 on principal and $20,000 for interest. What was the net income for the practice for the year?

_____

_____

_____

Income Statement Analysis

Chapter 7 discussed the use of ratios in the analysis of financial operations of the business reported on the balance sheet. Ratios are also an important tool in the analysis of the income statement. These ratios include the use of operating results in the income statement as well as information both from the balance sheet and available from other sources of the business. As with balance sheet analysis, ratios are most useful when changes are analyzed over time and when the ratio results of one business are compared to industry standards.

Liquidity Ratio: Days Cash Available Ratio

The **days cash available** ratio measures the number of days that cash and short-term investments would last, based on average daily expenses paid, as shown in Figure 7-4.

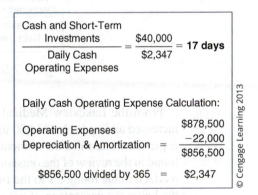

$$\frac{\text{Cash and Short-Term Investments}}{\text{Daily Cash Operating Expenses}} = \frac{\$40,000}{\$2,347} = \textbf{17 days}$$

Daily Cash Operating Expense Calculation:

$$\begin{array}{r}\text{Operating Expenses} \quad \$878,500 \\ \text{Depreciation \& Amortization} = \underline{-22,000} \\ \$856,500\end{array}$$

$$\$856,500 \text{ divided by } 365 = \$2,347$$

© Cengage Learning 2013

Figure 7-4 Days Available Cash Ratio

From the Lakeview Medical income statement (Figure 7-1), combined cash and short-term investments total $40,000. Total expenses of $878,500 are reduced by $22,000 for depreciation and amortization, and noncash expenses, and divided by 365 days in the year. Lakeview Medical has only 17 days' cash available, a fairly low level. A more optimal cash position would be 30 days' cash available; the indicator rising over time would tend to indicate a strengthening financial condition, unless caused by a onetime infusion of cash such as the sale of assets.

Case Study 7-1

Allied Hospitals owns and operates a number of hospitals in the American South. It is a publicly held corporation with stock traded on a major stock exchange. Tom Jackson is a stock analyst employed by a firm that monitors and rates stocks for investors. In Allied's annual financial report for December 31, 2020, the days available cash ratio was calculated at 62 days. At December 31, 2021, the ratio had declined to 28 days.

If you were in Mr. Jackson's position as analyst on Allied Hospitals stock, would you inform investors of this decline in the days cash available ratio?

Mr. Jackson made the decision that the decline in the days cash available ratio could be a significant issue and may affect the rating of the stock. Reviewing further, he found a note to the financial statements reporting that Allied had purchased an additional hospital in 2020 using a combination of cash and bank loans. Cash flow from operations continued to be strong during 2020, and the cash down payment on the hospital purchase would not impact their ability to pay their bills. Mr. Jackson's conclusion in his analyst report was that the decline in the days available cash ratio was not an indicator of declining financial performance. In this instance, the decline in the ratio only indicated the need to dig deeper into the financials. The change in the ratio did not indicate any financial difficulties.

Solvency Ratio: Debt Service Coverage Ratio

The **debt service coverage ratio** compares net income for the accounting period, generally 1 year, to the highest annual debt service obligation on outstanding debt.

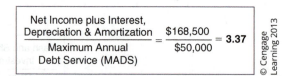

Figure 7-5 Debt Service Coverage Ratio

From the Lakeview Medical example in Figure 7-1, net income of $126,500 is increased adding back $22,000 in depreciation and amortization and $20,000 in interest expense to determine the numerator of the ratio. Maximum annual debt service may be found in the review of the outstanding debt instruments of the business, commonly summarized in the footnotes to the financial statements. The higher the results of this ratio, the lower the percentage of net income that must be used to service outstanding debt. The ratio will increase as profits increase, or debt service is reduced as debt is paid down. A decrease in this ratio is not always bad: the business may take on additional debt to finance revenue growth from the ability to perform more medical services.

Profit Level Ratios: Operating Margin and Return on Equity

The **operating margin** ratio is calculated by dividing net income by total revenues and is used to measure the efficiency of the operation.

$$\frac{\text{Net Income}}{\text{Total Revenues}} = \frac{\$126,500}{\$1,005,000} = 12.39\%$$

© Cengage Learning 2013

Figure 7-6 Operating Margin

This indicator has special importance in publicly traded for-profit medical businesses as profits generated by the business enhance stockholder equity and provide funds for dividends. Stock analysts will review increases in the operating margin over time and compare the operating margin to other competitors in the industry.

Profitability is always a concern of not-for-profit healthcare facilities, as too high a level of profit could mean that the facility could provide services to the community at lower rates, while losses would mean that the facility is required to use reserves to cover operating costs.

The **return on equity** ratio is calculated by dividing net income by the ownership equity (or net assets) of the organization.

$$\frac{\text{Net Income}}{\text{Owners' Equity}} = \frac{\$126,500}{\$419,100} = 30.18\%$$

© Cengage Learning 2013

Figure 7-7 Return on Equity

This ratio measures the efficiency of the operation to generate profit based on the investment made in the business. Successful organizations will improve this ratio over time.

Knowledge Check 7.3

1. In Figure 7-5, the debt service coverage ratio for Lakeview Medical Clinic was calculated at 3.37. Assume in the following year that Lakeview Medical's coverage ratio calculated at 1.50. What factors would you review to analyze the change in the debt service coverage ratio?

_____

_____

_____

2. In the 2020 financial statements of Northport Regional Hospital, the hospital reported $7,500,000 in total revenues and $285,000 in net income. The balance sheet at December 31, 2020, showed net assets of $4,200,000. Calculate both the operating margin ratio and the return on equity ratio for Northport.

_____

_____

_____

Key Concepts

- The income statement is the companion financial report to the balance sheet and shows the revenues, expenses, and net income of the operation.

- Net medical services revenues reflect revenues expected to be received by a medical facility after the full charges for services provided have been adjusted to the contract rates with healthcare insurance and government providers.

- Businesses are required to meet compliance requirements for minimum pay and overtime pay in the Fair Labor Standards Act (FLSA) of 1938 and state mandates.

- Net income represents the profitability of the operation and is the difference between revenues and expenses.

- Ratios are used to analyze business operations, to compare changes over time and between companies.

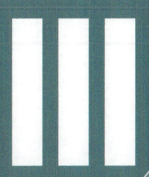

Section III

Healthcare Financial Management

Financial management includes several disciplines critical to the financial health of organizations. Section III includes discussions of budgeting, managing cash flow, investing available funds, borrowing, revenue cycle management, and issues involved with financial risk. The book concludes with a chapter on current advances in health information technology.

III

Healthcare Financial Management

Financial management includes several disciplines critical to the financial health of organizations. Section III includes discussions of budgeting, managing cash flow, investing available funds, borrowing, revenue cycle management, and issues involved with financial risk. The book concludes with a chapter on current advances in health information technology.

Budgets

Key Terms

Annual budget
Bottom-up budgeting
Break-even analysis
Budget
Budget amendment
Budget control
Capital budget
Cash budget
Chart of accounts
Encounters
Expenditure budget
Full-time equivalent (FTE)
Incremental budgeting
Operating budget
Revenue budget
Statistical budget
Top-down budgeting
Variance analysis
Zero-base budgeting (ZBB)

Chapter Objectives

After completing this chapter, readers should be able to:

- Explain the different types of budgets commonly used by healthcare facilities:

  1. Annual budget

  2. Authorized personnel budget

  3. Capital budget

  4. Expenditure budget

  5. Statistical budget

  6. Revenue budget

  7. Cash budget

- Compare top-down (authoritarian) budgeting and bottom-up (participatory) budgeting.

- Contrast incremental budgeting and zero-base budgeting.

- Discuss the process of amending the budget during the year, including the use of budget controls and budget amendments.

- Explain the budget development process for smaller medical facilities.

- Demonstrate the ability to perform break-even analysis.

Chapter Glossary

The **annual budget** of the organization combines the annual revenue budget and the annual expenditure budget.

Bottom-up budgeting is a participatory philosophy of budgeting, relying on unit managers to provide information on the unit's operational needs.

Break-even analysis is the budget mechanism that allows for the determination of the number of units of service that need to be provided to cover the organization's costs.

The **budget** is management's plan for a future period of time, expressed in dollars.

A **budget amendment** is the official approval to move funds from one budget line item to another.

Budget control is the level of flexibility provided to unit managers in using budgeted funds during the year.

The **capital budget** accounts for the major capital expenditures of the organization and is normally prepared to cover several budget years.

The **cash budget** projects revenues, expenditures, and cash flow on a monthly basis.

The **chart of accounts** is the listing of all line items used in the budget and accounting system to identify specific revenues and expenditures.

Encounters are the number of units of patient care provided by the medical facility.

Expenditure budget is the combination of approved operating budgets for the various departments, current year approved capital replacements and improvements, and cost items.

A **full-time equivalent (FTE)** position is based on one employee working 8 hours per day, 5 days per week, for 52 weeks per year.

Incremental budgeting starts with the current approved budget and adds funds for inflation and projected demands for service.

Operating budget, also commonly called the annual budget, combines the annual revenue budget and the annual expenditure budget.

The **revenue budget** starts with the projected revenues from patient care, based on the statistical budget (see the following term), and adds nonpatient revenues to project total revenues for the budget year.

The **statistical budget** projects patient care revenues based on units of service to be provided and established reimbursement rates.

Top-down budgeting places the control for the development of the budget in the hands of a limited number of individuals at the top management level of the organization.

Variance analysis is the periodic review of actual expenditures against the approved budget to determine compliance.

Zero-base budgeting (ZBB) requires that each unit manager responsible for a budget justify every item in the budget from a base of zero each budget year.

The units of service equation is:
Units of Service − Price × Volume = Fixed Costs + (Variable Cost per Unit × Volume)

The patient visit equation is:
Patient Visit − Fixed Costs/Revenue Per Visit − Variable Costs

Introduction

"If you have to forecast, forecast often."

(Edgar R. Fielder, www.brainyquote.com/quotes/authors/e/edgar_r_fielder.html)

"Yes, when we do a plan, it is at that moment static, because it shows what is assumed at the time you hit save. But life goes on, variables change, and your plans should change with it."

(Spivak, W., SBA Consulting Ltd, July 23, 2011; www.sbaconsulting.com/wordpress)

The **budget** is management's plan, expressed in dollars, for a future period of time. It reflects the medical facility's view of future demands for service and projections of financial resources available to provide services needed. Economic conditions can change rapidly, and these changing conditions require that the forecasts contained in the budget are updated regularly. This chapter will discuss the different types of budgets used by medical facilities, the process for developing the budgets, and how organizations respond to changing conditions.

Budgets become critically important in times of economic change. When revenues from providing medical services shrink, the budget provides detailed guidance on reducing costs to maintaining the solvency of the organization. As demand for services and related revenues increase, the budget allows for the allocation of these additional resources to meet the demand for services. The following example will illustrate this concept:

Example 8-1

A hospital is in a community where the dominant industry has experienced major layoffs and families are leaving the community in search of better job opportunities elsewhere. The local hospital has been forced to react to this loss of population. The revenue budget for the upcoming fiscal year has been reduced by lower patient care statistics. Forced to balance the budget at these lower revenue projections, the hospital has responded by eliminating salary increases, reducing the use of part-time employees, and deferring major investment in capital equipment.

In another state, a community has used tax breaks to attract a new business, promising to add 500 jobs to the local workforce. The chief executive officer of the local hospital in this growing community calls a planning meeting with senior management and the board of directors to discuss how they will respond to increases in demands for medical service. The revised budget provides for additional staff positions, increased overtime, and added funds for medical supplies. The projected higher revenues also provide for funds to replace old and obsolete equipment while maintaining a balanced budget.

The Operating Budget

The **annual budget**, also commonly known as the **operating budget** of the organization, combines the annual revenue budget and the annual expenditure budget. The **expenditure budget** for the organization is the combination of approved operating budgets for the various departments, current year approved capital replacements and improvements, and cost items such as annual depreciation and amortization not accounted for in specific departments. The difference between the projected annual operating revenues and the expected expenditures for the year yields the profit or loss from annual operations.

When staff members talk about "the budget," the document referred to is the annual operating budget for their work unit. Commonly heard statements are, "I'm sorry, you cannot attend that conference because it is not in the budget," and "We're almost out of our supply budget, so we'll have to be more careful for the rest of the year."

The annual budget in Figure 8-1, also called the operating budget, displays how the annual revenue budget and annual expenditure budget impact a healthcare facility's overall budget.

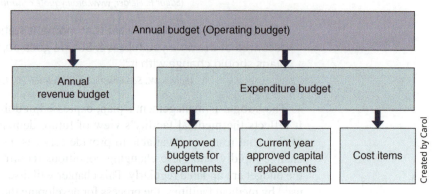

Figure 8-1 Annual Budget

Figure 8-2 shows the completed base operating budget for nursing services in the hospital. This completed budget is the result of the nurse manager working with the hospital's finance department to prepare a budget based on financial resources that are expected to be available in the upcoming calendar year. While all budgeting formats are different, that is, structured to meet the needs of an individual organization, it is common to see operating budgets broken down into a limited number of groups of individual line items. Line items are individual cost areas and are commonly combined into major categories. In the example shown in Figure 8-2, the budgeting system uses three major headings of costs.

DEPARTMENT OPERATING BUDGET

Account Code	Account Description	Actual 2008	Actual 2009	Budget 2010	2010 6 Months	2010 Projected	2011 Budget
SALARIES & BENEFITS:							
	Salaries-Full-Time	725,331	762,348	810,000	345,923	750,000	826,200
	Salaries-Part-Time	52,878	38,758	40,000	62,743	88,000	60,000
	Overtime	12,878	15,980	15,000	12,858	20,000	15,000
	Shift Differential	88,678	92,567	100,000	44,756	90,000	102,000
	FICA	68,085	71,489	75,000	35,685	72,500	76,000
	Health Insurance	55,875	60,923	65,000	29,371	62,000	71,500
	Pension	38,945	40,244	48,600	19,867	44,200	49,500
	SUB-TOTAL	**1,042,670**	**1,082,309**	**1,153,600**	**551,203**	**1,126,700**	**1,200,200**
OPERATING EXPENSES:							
	Office Supplies	2,379	3,453	3,000	812	2,000	2,200
	Patient Care Supplies	29,823	31,872	33,000	16,872	35,000	35,900
	Travel & Training	5,624	6,298	6,500	1,982	6,500	6,500
	Memberships	1,850	1,975	2,000	1,550	2,000	2,000
	Equipment Repair	9,824	2,976	3,500	1,793	2,500	3,500
	Rentals & Leases	2,369	2,652	2,750	1,872	3,000	3,200
	Miscellaneous	192	347	300	92	200	300
	SUB-TOTAL	**52,061**	**49,573**	**51,050**	**24,973**	**51,200**	**53,600**
	ALLOCATED COSTS	**110,242**	**117,126**	**125,000**	**62,500**	**125,000**	**133,000**
	TOTAL	**1,204,973**	**1,249,008**	**1,329,650**	**638,676**	**1,302,900**	**1,386,800**

Note that the department operating budget does not provide funds for the replacement of capital equipment. Those costs are included in a separate capital budget.

Figure 8-2 An Example of a Completed Operating Budget for a Nursing Department

© Cengage Learning 2013

Salaries and Benefits

The budget for each department for salaries and benefits is traditionally developed by the finance and human resources staffs, accounting for projections for available funding for the year and competitive pressures from other employers in attracting and retaining quality staff. In Figure 8-2, the financial forecast is for a continued tight economy with minimal inflation for the next year and no major wage pressures from other local employers. A retirement plan where the employer promises to make a guaranteed contribution to each employee's individual retirement account is referred to as a **defined contribution retirement plan**. A retirement plan where the employee is promised monthly retirement income based on a formula of salary and years of service is a **defined benefit retirement plan**. The hospital used as an example in Figure 8-2 has a defined contribution plan for employees.

Operating Expenses

For the nursing services cost center, the largest cost area under operating expenses is the purchase of patient care supplies. The hospital's purchasing manager reports that costs have increased for the purchase of these items over the past year and that prices are likely to remain high in the upcoming months. The budget office has responded to these cost increases by providing a 5 percent increase in operating expenses to the nursing department for a new total of $53,600 for the 2020 budget. Other cost items within operating expenses are the costs of maintaining continuing education requirements, equipment rentals and leases, and miscellaneous costs of running the department for the year. The nurse manager has the responsibility of allocating the $53,600 for operating expenses to support the department most effectively for the upcoming year.

Allocated Costs

All medical facilities have functions that are required by the organization but that do not bring in revenues. In the budget example in Figure 8-2, the costs of central maintenance and the payment for utilities and insurance are budgeted in a separate department, with the costs of operating that department recovered by allocating those costs to revenue-producing departments such as nursing, surgery, and the emergency room. In this example, the nursing department will contribute $133,000 to support those centralized costs.

The operating budget is the budget most familiar to unit managers and their staffs. The unit manager will most likely be heavily involved in the annual budget preparation process and will be provided monthly updates from the accounting system that will allow the manager to track compliance with the budget throughout the year. The operating budgets for each individual work unit are combined into the master operating budget for the healthcare facility. The master operating budget of the organization will include any areas of expense, such as depreciation of capital assets that are not accounted for within department operating budgets.

Developing the Operating Budget

The hospital has adopted the calendar year as their fiscal year. Soon after the end of June, halfway through the fiscal year, the hospital's finance department prepares draft budget forms and provides them to the managers of each of the hospital's work units. This report shows actual results for the previous two fiscal years, the current year budget, and actual results for the first 6 months of the current year. The responsibility of the nurse manager is to complete the 2019 projected column based on experience of the first 6 months and funding requirements for the upcoming 6 months.

DEPARTMENT OPERATING BUDGET

Account Code	Account Description	Actual 2017	Actual 2018	Budget 2019	2019 6 Months	2019 Projected	2020 Budget
SALARIES & BENEFITS:							
	Salaries-Full-Time	725,331	762,348	810,000	345,923		826,200
	Salaries-Part-Time	52,878	38,758	40,000	62,743		60,000
	Overtime	12,878	15,980	15,000	12,858		15,000
	Shift Differential	88,678	92,567	100,000	44,756		102,000
	FICA	68,085	71,489	75,000	35,685		76,000
	Health Insurance	55,875	60,923	65,000	29,371		71,500
	Pension	38,945	40,244	48,600	19,867		49,500
	SUB-TOTAL	**1,042,670**	**1,082,309**	**1,153,600**	**551,203**	**–**	**1,200,200**
OPERATING EXPENSES:							
	Office Supplies	2,379	3,453	3,000	812		
	Patient Care Supplies	29,823	31,872	33,000	16,872		
	Travel & Training	5,624	6,298	6,500	1,982		
	Memberships	1,850	1,975	2,000	1,550		
	Equipment Repair	9,824	2,976	3,500	1,793		
	Rentals & Leases	2,369	2,652	2,750	1,872		
	Miscellaneous	192	347	300	92		
	SUB-TOTAL	**52,061**	**49,573**	**51,050**	**24,973**	**–**	**53,600**
	ALLOCATED COSTS	**110,242**	**117,126**	**125,000**	**62,500**	**125,000**	**133,000**
	TOTAL	**1,204,973**	**1,249,008**	**1,329,650**	**638,676**	**125,000**	**1,386,800**

© Cengage Learning 2013

Figure 8-3 An Example of an Operating Budget Draft for a Nursing Department

Each department manager is asked to project salaries and benefits for the entire fiscal year based on experience in the first 6 months. This information is used by the budget office to forecast operating results for the entire facility for the year. Note in Figure 8-3 that the nursing department lost several full-time staff members to resignation and were forced to make up staff hours with a combination of part-time employees and overtime. While those two line items will be over budget for the year, underspending in full-time salaries keeps the work unit within budget. The nurse manager will need to project when the full-time positions will be filled to complete the salaries and benefits section of the 2019 projected budget.

In the operating expenses section, the nurse manager will use historical cost data to project operating expenses for the full fiscal year 2019. Hospital management has agreed to a 5 percent increase in operating expenses for fiscal year 2020, providing the nursing department with an operating expenses budget of $53,600. The nurse manager will spread that amount, as needed, between the various line items within the budget section.

No action is required from the nurse manager on the allocated costs section. That information is completed by the finance department.

Comprehension Check 8.1

1. The expenditure budget is comprised of what three types of items?

2. When staff members talk about "the budget" in a healthcare facility, they are referring to which budget?

3. What is the annual budget commonly known as?

The Authorized Personnel Budget

Regular full-time staffing for the healthcare facility is based on **full-time equivalent (FTE)** positions. The standard was developed based on one employee job position requiring the employee in the position to work 8 hours per day, 5 days per week, for 52 weeks per year—an annual total of 2,080 hours:

8 hours/day × 5 days/week × 52 weeks/year = 2,080 hours per full-time position

The standard for an 8-hour day, 5 days per week may work well for a factory with a fixed 8-hour shift. Healthcare facilities will adjust the FTE calculation to meet the staffing requirements of a 24-hour daily operation. The 2,080-hour total is derived from wage and hour laws requiring the payment of overtime to nonexempt employees working over 40 hours per week. Wage and hour laws are mandated in each state. Overtime required for work in excess of 40 hours per week is the most common; however, some states require overtime pay for work over 8 hours in a day.

The statistical budget, discussed later on in the chapter, projects the units of service to be provided during the budget year. These service units provide the workload of the organization and are the basis for the staffing needs. When service units are projected to increase, staffing in the form of additional FTEs may also need to be increased. Declines in projected service units may result in a lower FTE budget.

In Figure 8-4, nursing has authorized full-time staffing of 19 positions, each working 40-hour work weeks. The same formula is used to develop the FTE count for any permanent part-time positions. For 2010, nursing was authorized 1.8 FTE part-time positions for total available staff hours of 72 hours per week (1.8 FTE × 40 hours = 72). The nurse manager can use different employees for different numbers of hours so long as the total hours worked by part-time employees does not exceed a weekly average of 72 hours throughout the budget year. This authorization provides the flexibility to react to higher or lower workloads at certain times of the year. For 2011, the authorization for part-time employees was increased to 2.2 FTE, or an average of 88 hours per week. For both full- and part-time employees, salaries and hourly wages have been determined by the human resources department.

DEPARTMENT: NURSING SERVICES			
	2010 FTE	2010 FTE	2011 Salary
Nurse Manager	1.0	1.0	82,300
Registered Nurse (RN)	7.0	7.0	362,400
Licensed Practical Nurse (LPN)	4.0	4.0	167,200
Nursing Assistant: Full-Time	4.0	4.0	122,600
Patient Care Technician	3.0	3.0	91,700
FULL-TIME FTE:	**19.0**	**19.0**	**826,200**
Nursing Assistant: Part-Time	1.8	2.2	60,000
PART-TIME FTE:	**1.8**	**2.2**	**60,000**

The authorized personnel budget provides the unit manager with the maximum amount of staffing approved to meet the department's goals and objectives.

© Cengage Learning 2013

Figure 8-4 Authorized Personnel Budget for a Nursing Department

In most healthcare organizations, salaries and benefits are the largest components of the annual budget. Too few employees may result in less than optimal patient care; too many employees may result in overcharging for medical services. **Benchmarking** measures the number of employee positions for a specific function or activity against established industry standards. An effective introduction to benchmarking in healthcare can be found at PubMed, a website developed by the U.S. National Library of Medicine of the National Institutes of Health (NIH; **Making the numbers work for you: Establishing effective compensation**; www.ncbi.nlm.nih.gov/pubmed).

With the complexities involved in benchmarking, many organizations use the assistance of outside consultants.

Capital Budget

The operating budget and the authorized personnel budget are prepared each year and cover a single fiscal year. The **capital budget**, as the name implies, is used to schedule the purchase of assets that will have a long useful life. The first step in the process is agreement on the definition of what purchases will be considered capital and what purchases will be expensed. A common working definition is that to be considered a capital acquisition, the asset must have an original purchase price in excess of $2,500 and have a useful life of more than 1 year. The $2,500 threshold is commonly used and agrees with Medicare accounting requirements. Any purchase that does not meet the definition will be expensed in the year purchased and charged to the operating budget under a heading such as "Office Supplies."

The second step in the development of the capital budget is determining the number of years to be covered; 5 to 10 years is common. Once decisions have been made on the first two steps, the budget office will meet with unit managers to review the detailed listing of assets owned by the medical facility and assigned to each unit. Each of these assets will become obsolete or worn out and will need to be replaced at a point in the future. The concept of accounting for this loss in value through depreciation was previously discussed in the chapter on the balance sheet. If the asset will need to be replaced within the time frame of the capital budget, the cost of the replacement will need to be budgeted. Two items become important in completing this step:

1. The cost of the asset at a future point in time

2. The year that the asset needs to be replaced

The budget office will combine the replacement schedules for each work unit into a master capital expenditure budget for the healthcare facility. The next logical question is, "How does the business pay for all of this?" The financing of the capital budget will come from two primary sources:

1. **Internally generated funds**. The income statement of the healthcare facility shows a charge for the depreciation of assets that serves to reduce net income. Depreciation is not a cash item; however, assuming that the facility operates at better than break-even net income, cash is available for the replacement of assets. As an example, a small medical practice has total revenues for the year of $1,000,000 and expenditures for salaries and operating expenses of $950,000. The $50,000 balance equals the annual charge for depreciation, bringing net income to zero. However, assuming that items such as accounts receivable and accounts payable did not change from the prior year-end, $50,000 has been generated during the course of the year that can be used for capital replacement.

2. **Borrowing**. When funds generated internally are not sufficient to cover the costs of assets that need to be replaced, the second option is borrowing. Financing capital acquisitions will be discussed in the chapter on borrowing and the time value of money. Borrowing is an acceptable alternative when the revenues of the healthcare facility are sufficient to cover the annual debt service costs.

The capital budget is updated each year, with the capital expenditures budgeted in the first year of the long-range capital budget included in the combined budget of the facility for the upcoming fiscal year. All new capital acquisitions will immediately begin to lose value through depreciation. Charges for depreciation on new assets will need to be accounted for in the organization's annual operating budget.

Statistical and Revenue Budgets

The operating budgets, authorized personnel budgets, and capital budgets, as discussed previously, deal with the expenses of running the healthcare organization. For the organization to remain financially viable, sufficient revenues need to be earned to offset these expenses.

Before Medicare and the widespread use of group health insurance, projecting revenue was a reasonably simple task. A hospital had a certain number of beds and charged one rate for a private room and a different rate for a semiprivate room. The number of beds times the daily rate for each, times 365 days, times the projected occupancy factor yielded revenues from inpatient room charges. Today, private-pay patients are a small percentage of total patients. Government programs and a wide variety of group health insurers cover most of the patients. Each government program and insurance provider will have their individual schedules for reimbursement of hospital charges.

The **statistical budget** projects patient care revenues based on units of service to be provided, weights assigned to each service, and applies reimbursement rates to determine net medical service revenues.

To develop the statistical budget, the budget office will start with a listing of each service that the hospital is compensated for. Figure 8-5 is simplified to show only patient admissions and follow-up care. **Encounters**, the number of units of service to be provided for patient care, are estimated based on historical activity and understanding of the current economic environment. Each type of patient encounter is given an assigned weight. The assigned weight is a multiple of a base charge for service. In Figure 8-5, admissions are assigned a weight factor of 5.0, meaning that the hospital's standard fee is five times greater than a base service charge. Follow-up visits have an assigned weight of 1.5. Multiplying the number of projected encounters by the assigned weight provides the number of weighted encounters.

The **revenue budget** uses as its basis data that have been developed through the statistical budget. See Figure 8-6 for a sample revenue budget.

The number of weighted encounters from the statistical budget becomes the first column in the revenue budget. The hospital has determined that the dollar value per weight will be $100. That number will increase as the hospital's costs of providing service increase due to higher labor costs, operating expenses, and requirements for new technology. Multiplying the number of projected weighted encounters by the $100 value per weight yields gross medical services revenues.

Group health insurance providers have negotiated contracts with the hospital that establish fee schedules providing reimbursement for medical services at a rate less than the hospital's full-services fees. Medicare and Medicaid have their own fee schedules, also less than the hospital's full-service fees. The discounts from the full fee schedule result in contractual adjustments that serve to reduce gross medical service revenues to net medical service revenues.

STATISTICAL BUDGET
Month of April 20XX

	Encounters	Assigned Weight	Weighted Encounters
Employment Based			
Admissions	300	5.0	1,500
Follow-up care	1,200	1.5	1,800
Medicare			
Admissions	600	5.0	3,000
Follow-up care	1,900	1.5	2,850
Medicaid			
Admissions	100	5.0	500
Follow-up care	250	1.5	375
Private Pay			
Admissions	50	5.0	250
Follow-up care	100	1.5	150
MONTH TOTALS	**4,500**		**10,425**

Defined above, encounters are the number of units of patient care provided.

© Cengage Learning 2013

Figure 8-5 An Example of a Statistical Budget Used to Determine Patient Care Revenues Based on Units of Services

The revenue budget in Figure 8-6 covers the month of April 2020. The same process will be performed for all other months of the year to determine annual patient care revenues. Added to that total of patient care revenues are any sources of nonpatient care revenues. Nonpatient care revenues can come from a variety of sources. Some hospitals will have an in-house gift and flower shop and may operate a pharmacy. Many nonprofit hospitals will court donor revenues to support their operations and will actively seek governmental grants. Also included in the revenue budget is any

REVENUE BUDGET
Month of April 20XX

	Weighted Encounters	Value per Weight	Gross Medical Revenues	Discount	Contractual Adjustments	Net Medical Revenues
Employment Based						
Admissions	1,500	$100.00	$150,000.00	40%	$60,000.00	$90,000.00
Follow-up care	1,800	$100.00	180,000.00	40%	72,000.00	108,000.00
Medicare						
Admissions	3,000	$100.00	300,000.00	50%	150,000.00	150,000.00
Follow-up care	2,850	$100.00	285,000.00	50%	142,500.00	142,500.00
Medicaid						
Admissions	500	$100.00	50,000.00	60%	30,000.00	20,000.00
Follow-up care	375	$100.00	37,500.00	60%	22,500.00	15,000.00
Private Pay						
Admissions	250	$100.00	25,000.00	–	–	25,000.00
Follow-up care	150	$100.00	15,000.00	–	–	15,000.00
MONTH TOTALS	**10,425**		**$1,042,500.00**		**$477,000.00**	**$565,500.00**

© Cengage Learning 2013

Figure 8-6 An Sample Revenue Budget Worksheet

borrowing required to support the budgeted expenditures in the capital budget. The total of all patient care revenues and nonpatient care revenues becomes the total of the revenue budget.

Comprehension Check 8.2

1. Which type of budget allows for new assets to be purchased based on prior assets reaching the useful life of operation?

2. Which type of budget projects patient care revenues based on unit of service to be provided and weights assigned to each service, and applies reimbursement rates to determine net medical service revenues?

3. Which two areas are the largest components of the annual budget?

Knowledge Check

8.1

1. Explain the key difference between the operating budget and the capital budget.

_____

_____

_____

2. Define full-time equivalents (FTEs).

_____

_____

_____

3. The medical records office of a healthcare facility is budgeted with four full-time positions and 1.2 FTE part-time positions. For how many hours per year can the medical records supervisor use part-time employees?

_____

_____

_____

4. A hospital has 100 beds in 50 semiprivate rooms. Average occupancy over the past several years has been 70 percent. Determine the number of projected encounters using the 70 percent occupancy factor. Determine the number of weighted encounters under the assumption that the assigned weight is 4.0.

_____

_____

_____

5. Using the weighted encounters in question 4, determine the revenue budget for the hospital using the assumptions that the value per weighted encounter is $100 and that all patients have employment-based healthcare insurance with a discount factor of 40 percent.

_____

_____

_____

The Cash Budget

The revenue budget and the expenditure budget are prepared for the full fiscal year. For almost all medical facilities, patient care volumes are not spread equally over the 12 months. They will be busier at certain times of year than at others. Compounding the variances in volumes of patient care is the lag time between patient care and reimbursement for services provided. The medical facility will have certain times of the year that are busier than others, requiring overtime to be paid and additional hours worked by part-time employees. Those costs are paid with the current payrolls prior to reimbursement being received. The **cash budget** starts with the annual budget for total revenues and total expenditures, and based on historical data, divides the budget into monthly columns. Each month will have either positive or negative cash flow. Analysis of the cash budget will inform the finance department of the level of cash reserves required to pay current expenditures and avoid the need for short-term borrowing. Sophisticated cash budgeting systems can be used to analyze cash flow on a daily or weekly basis in addition to the monthly cash budget shown in Figure 8-7.

	MARCH	OCTOBER
Blue Cross/Others Insurance	145,000	210,000
Medicare/Medicaid	165,000	225,000
Private Pay	40,000	45,000
Miscellaneous Receipts	5,000	5,000
CASH RECEIPTS	**355,000**	**485,000**
Personnel Costs	150,000	170,000
Payments to Suppliers	25,000	30,000
Capital Assets Purchased	10,000	40,000
Debt Service	200,000	200,000
CASH DISBURSEMENTS	**385,000**	**440,000**
MONTHLY CASH FLOW	**(30,000)**	**45,000**

© Cengage Learning 2013

Figure 8-7 An Example of a Monthly Cash Budget

Example 8-2

Great Plains Medical is located in Nebraska. The town's primary businesses support the surrounding agricultural areas. A sizable percentage of the town's population is older adults, residing here from spring through fall and spending the winter months in warmer climates. The medical facility sees a large increase in patient load during the fall months from farm accidents when the crops are harvested, medical needs of the families of migrant agricultural workers, and the normal injuries associated with

high school football. The winter months are much slower, with farmland dormant and older adults gone for the coldest months. The cash budget in Figure 8-7 shows the financial impact on two selected months during the facility's budget year: March and October. George Trafford is the financial manager for the medical facility and has developed this cash budget for the upcoming fiscal year. Mr. Trafford reviews the cash budget with his boss, identifying those months where the facility will expect to have to finance negative cash flow for a period of time.

Knowledge Check 8.2

1. What is the purpose of the cash budget?

_____

_____

_____

2. In Example 8-2, the Great Plains Medical facility had budgeted negative cash flow for the month of March of $30,000. In the full year cash budget, February had budgeted negative cash flow of $47,500 and April was negative $25,000. January, including insurance payments from care provided near the end of the prior year, was budgeted at break-even cash flow. All of the other months for the year were budgeted with positive cash flow. At the end of the calendar year on December 31, what is the minimum level of cash reserves necessary to pay operating costs of the facility without using borrowing?

_____

_____

_____

Putting It All Together

The discussion earlier in this chapter covered each of the major budgets needed to effectively manage the financial operations of a healthcare facility. Each of these budgets forms a part of the overall budgeting process shown in Figure 8-8.

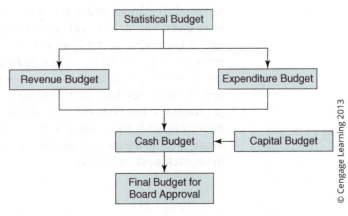

Figure 8-8 A Flow Chart of the Budgeting Process

The statistical budget comes first, projecting the demand for services. Using that demand for services, projections are made for revenues from medical services. Other sources of revenues are added to determine total projected revenues. Again, based on the demand for service, the expense budget is prepared to identify the costs associated with personnel needs of the organization and other operating expenses to meet the service demands. The capital budget is prepared, and the first year of that budget is included in the annual budgeting process. The cash budget is then prepared to determine any potential need for short-term borrowing to finance operations.

Budget Philosophies

- Top-down budgeting places control of the budgeting process in upper-level management.

- Bottom-up budgeting includes all levels of management in the budgeting process.

- Incremental budgeting begins with the current approved budget and adjusts funding to account for inflation and service demands.

- Zero-base budgeting requires all managers to justify all areas of expense for their areas of responsibility, with no funding guaranteed.

Top-down Budgeting

Top-down budgeting places the control for the development of the budget in the hands of a limited number of individuals at the top management level of the organization. Managers in the finance and executive offices will prepare the budget, projecting the needs of the various work units of the organization, and present the budget to the lower-level managers and supervisors when completed. Unit managers, directly responsible for the effective operations of the unit, have minimal input into the process. This budgeting philosophy has also been referred to as **authoritarian budgeting**. Maintaining control at the top level of the organization allows the budgeting process to move more quickly and smoothly.

Bottom-up Budgeting

Bottom-up budgeting provides for the direct input of unit managers into the budgeting process. These unit managers are the individuals most familiar with the operations of the unit and their budget needs to continue to provide effective service delivery. Bottom-up budgeting is also called **participatory budgeting**. This type of budgeting will serve to promote better understanding of the organization's goals and financial limitations and can enhance the communication and cooperation between work units. The major drawback to this level of participation in the budgeting process lies in the budgeting philosophies of individual unit managers. The food services manager may well be very conscientious and conservative in budgeting, requesting only those budget funds that have been proven necessary to run the unit. The radiology manager may take the budgeting approach that since management cuts her budget request every year, she will add in extra budget requests to allow for cuts while protecting funds for essential services. The budget manager of the facility needs to be aware of these differences and prepare a consolidated budget for the organization that treats each work unit fairly.

Incremental Budgeting

"How much more money do you need to run your unit next year?" **Incremental budgeting** starts with the authorized budget for the current fiscal year and adds additional funds to account for the effects of inflation and projected demands for service in the upcoming budget year. The positive side to incremental budgeting is that it makes the budgeting process for unit managers a simple procedure. The manager knows the current line item budget and the amount that has been expended to date. All that is needed is to project next year's costs for operating the unit in the same manner as it currently runs. The review of the proposed budget for the next year then centers only on the new costs added to the budget, not on the necessity of the funding level in the current budget. The obvious downside to incremental budgeting is the assumption that all funds budgeted in the current year are being used in a prudent and necessary manner. Even with this major flaw, incremental budgeting is the system used in most organizations.

Zero-Base Budgeting (ZBB)

"Zero-Based Budgeting (ZBB) is an approach to budgeting that starts from the premise that no costs or activities should be factored into the plans for the coming budget period, just because they figured in the costs or activities for the current or previous periods. Rather, everything that is to be included in the budget must be considered and justified."

(The Chartered Institute of Public Finance and Accountancy; www.cipfa.org.uk/pt/download/zero_based_budgeting_briefing.pdf.)

Zero-base budgeting (ZBB) attempts to address the weaknesses in incremental budgeting by requiring that all work units justify their budgets from a base of zero. Every position needs to be justified every year and every expenditure line item is analyzed first to determine the necessity of the cost and potential ways to reduce spending if that cost cannot be eliminated. Advances in technology have provided numerous opportunities to reduce costs. Training available over the Internet can be used in lieu of expensive travel to a remote city for required continuing education. A sophisticated telephone answering system can eliminate the need for full-time staff members to answer phones and direct calls. ZBB forces all managers to look for these types of alternatives when preparing their budgets. ZBB does not come without a downside: justifying every position and every line item every year is a time-consuming process and will tend to generate massive volumes of paperwork to be reviewed by the budget office and management. Key issues may be lost in the process.

Some organizations have chosen to combine incremental budgeting with zero-base budgeting as a satisfactory middle ground. ZBB is required of work units on a rotating basis. In 1 year, full budget justification is required from one or more work units, with the rest of the organization using incremental budgeting. The following year, different work units will use ZBB, and the cycle will be continued until all work units have been subjected to ZBB.

Comprehension Check 8.3

1. Cindy Ventrew is a unit manager at All-In-One medical facility. She has been with the facility for more 10 years. She appreciates feeling valued at the medical facility because, as a unit manager, she can give input into the budget of the facility. Which type of budget philosophy is All-In-One medical facility utilizing?

2. An x-ray technologist works for a well-known research hospital. Whenever he asks his manager about going to conferences out of state, his manager will suggest virtual conferences because of the cost factors on the budget. Which type of budget philosophy is the hospital using?

3. At Mellowwood Hospital, the executive team is responsible for preparing the budget. Once completed, the unit managers and supervisors are given the budget with no input from the management team. Which type of budget philosophy is the hospital using?

Knowledge Check

8.3

1. Compare and contrast top-down (authoritarian) budgeting and bottom-up (participatory) budgeting, showing the strengths and weaknesses of each.

_____

_____

_____

2. Explain incremental budgeting and zero-base budgeting. What are the advantages and disadvantages of each?

_____

_____

_____

The Final Step: Balancing the Budget

The end result of the budgeting process is always to maintain the financial viability of the organization; operating revenues for the year should be sufficient to cover operating expenditures and provide for debt service payments and capital investment for the replacement of aged or obsolete equipment. For all medical facilities, revenues are limited by government reimbursement rates, group health contracts, and requirements to provide uncompensated care. Using the revenue projections as a ceiling for expenditures, budget managers have the responsibility of preparing expenditure budgets within those limited resources but still provide sufficient funds to properly provide patient care services.

There is always temptation during the process to balance the budget to take the easy way out. If senior officials and unit managers are comfortable with the proposed expenditure budget but projected revenues will not support that level of expenditure, the easy way is to budget for increased patient visits for the upcoming budget year. The budget is balanced; however, the problem has only been pushed out to the new budget year, when monthly reviews indicate that revenues are not reaching the budgeted levels and require midyear budget cuts. The prudent approach is to start with a realistic revenue budget and make adjustments (budget cuts) to the expenditure budget until the budget is in balance.

Midcourse Corrections

The financial statements of the healthcare organization provide the historical perspective on the financial operations of the organization. They look back at what has happened and provide a clear record for the informed reader. The purpose of budgeting is based on projections rather than actual experience. These projections are estimates only and will always be subject to adjustment as the organization progresses through the budget year. The process of reviewing actual experience during the year compared to the projections contained in the approved budget is variance analysis.

In Figure 8-9, the nurse manager has received the operations report for the first 6 months of the budget year, compared to the actual experience of the prior year and the approved budget for the current year. Soon after the start of the budget year, two nurses resigned and the recruitment process for their replacement has proven to be lengthy. To maintain services, the nurse manager approved overtime for remaining staff and asked part-time employees to work additional hours to provide adequate coverage. While the nursing department continues to operate within budget, full-time salaries are projected to end the year under budget due to the staff vacancies, while both part-time salaries and overtime will be overspent for the year.

DEPARTMENT OPERATING BUDGET

Account Code	Account Description	Actual 2009	Budget 2010	2010 6 Months
	SALARIES & BENEFITS:			
	Salaries-Full-Time	762,348	810,000	345,923
	Salaries-Part-Time	38,758	40,000	62,743
	Overtime	15,980	15,000	12,858
	Shift Differential	92,567	100,000	44,756
	FICA	71,489	75,000	35,685
	Health Insurance	60,923	65,000	29,371
	Pension	40,244	48,600	19,867
	SUB-TOTAL	**1,082,309**	**1,153,600**	**551,203**
	OPERATING EXPENSES:			
	Office Supplies	3,453	3,000	812
	Patient Care Supplies	31,872	33,000	16,872
	Travel & Training	6,298	6,500	1,982
	Memberships	1,975	2,000	1,550
	Equipment Repair	2,976	3,500	1,793
	Rentals & Leases	2,652	2,750	1,872
	Miscellaneous	347	300	92
	SUB-TOTAL	**49,573**	**51,050**	**24,973**
	ALLOCATED COSTS	**117,126**	**125,000**	**62,500**
	TOTAL	**1,249,008**	**1,329,650**	**638,676**

© Cengage Learning 2013

Figure 8-9 Example of a Variance Analysis Comparing the Projected to the Actual

Budget Control

Budget control is the level of flexibility provided to unit managers in using budgeted funds during the year. The most stringent level of budget control is **line item control**. This control policy prohibits a unit manager from spending funds from any line item where the expenditure would exceed the budget for that individual line item.

The other end of the extreme is **department budget control**, where the unit manager is authorized to use any available funds within the total budget for the year, regardless of whether any individual line items are overspent. A middle ground is **section control**, providing that individual line items may be overspent, but the actual expenditures within the subtotal for each major section of the budget must remain within budget. Healthcare facilities will adopt a budget control philosophy based on personal preference and experience.

Budget Amendments

A **budget amendment** is the official approval to move funds from one budget line item to another. As medical organizations grow larger and their budgets become more complex, a structured process to amend the budget is needed. The form will generally be initiated by the unit manager, be approved by the budget office, and receive final approval from the executive level of the organization. In some instances, approval of the board of directors will be required. Using the example in Figure 8-10, the nurse manager would determine from human resources when the vacant nursing positions would be filled and project the continued need for overtime and use of part-time employees. A budget amendment form would be prepared by the nurse manager to add funds to both the part-time salaries and overtime line items, reducing the line item for full-time salaries by the combined amount of the increases. The subtotal for salaries and benefits has not changed, nor has the total department budget. Figure 8-10 shows a sample budget amendment form.

ST. REGIS HOSPITAL
BUDGET AMENDMENT

	ACCOUNT CODE	DESCRIPTION	AMOUNT
FROM:	_____	_____	_____
	_____	_____	_____
	_____	_____	_____
TO:	_____	_____	_____
	_____	_____	_____
	_____	_____	_____
	_____	_____	_____

JUSTIFICATION: _____
_____
_____

APPROVED:
_____   _____   _____
UNIT   BUDGET   EXECUTIVE
MANAGER   MANAGER   OFFICER

© Cengage Learning 2013

Figure 8-10 A Sample Budget Amendment Form

Knowledge Check

8.4

1. Because of crop failures in Europe, American farm equipment manufacturers are gearing up production to meet expected increased demand. The manufacturing facility in Smithville, Georgia, is adding a second shift and hiring new workers. Smithville Community Hospital operates on a calendar-year budget. By midyear, the hospital is seeing a substantial increase in patient visits, and the operating units in the hospital are experiencing needs for higher use of overtime and part-time employees, exceeding budgeted funds. You are the budget manager for Smithville Community Hospital. What budget amendments would you recommend to both hospital management and the board of directors?

_____

_____

_____

2. The largest employer in Jones Corner, Indiana, builds travel trailers and has been battered by the current recession, reducing employment to meet the loss in sales volume. A number of families have moved away to seek employment elsewhere. Physicians Hospital in Jones Corner has experienced reductions in patient visits, and the hospital's budget manager is projecting that the hospital will not meet revenue or cash budget. You are the administrator for Physicians Hospital. You meet with the budget manager to formulate a plan of action to take to the board of directors. What budget amendments will you consider to meet the loss in revenues?

_____

_____

Budgeting for Smaller Medical Facilities

Even in a successful medical facility, budgeting provides an essential early warning system of financial problems that may lie ahead. When revenues are not reaching the levels projected in the budget, the physician and practice manager can look for ways to increase revenues or take steps necessary to ensure that expenses are reduced to meet the lower revenue levels. Expenditure line items that seem to be unusually high can be reviewed to determine the cause of the overspending and steps taken to control costs. The budgeting system will also serve to uncover employee embezzlement early. Detecting these problems as they arise will allow the practice to take corrective action before the problems become critical.

Case Study 8-1

Margaret Coleman, practice manager for Dr. Corwin, was meeting with coworkers and commented: "I know the practice should have a budget, but I never seem to be able to find the time to do it." Dr. Corwin has been in practice for a number of years, and the practice produces revenues sufficient to pay all of the business expenses and provides a comfortable lifestyle for the doctor and his family. The practice uses accounting software; Ms. Coleman has been trained on the software and knows how to manage it to add new revenue and expense account codes. What steps should Ms. Coleman take to develop a budget for the practice?

Five Steps to Developing an Effective Budget

The development of an annual budget takes information that is available in the financial records of the organization and organizes that data into a format that may be used to forecast future revenues and expenditures. The process of budget development consists of the following five steps:

1. Prepare a chart of accounts.

2. Track historical revenues and costs.

3. Benchmark costs.

4. Build the annual budget.

5. Review the monthly budget.

Step One: Prepare a Chart of Accounts

In accounting, the **chart of accounts** is a list of the names of income (revenue), expense (what the business spends), liability (what the business owes), and asset (what the business owns) accounts that a company uses in maintaining their books in a general ledger. The chart of accounts is set up by finance at the start of the business. Reference numbers are used to help classify the accounts by type. For example, in a hospital, each nursing unit will have a reference number. The chart organizes and tracks all of the business activities. Reports can then be easily generated in a logical sequence to track the financial history and progress of the business.

The accounting system already tracks expenditures by line item, and this list forms the basis of the chart of accounts. Items may be added or deleted based on the specific needs of the practice. Figure 8-11 is a chart of accounts for a single physician medical practice.

The chart of accounts can be as simple or as detailed as needed to provide the needed financial information. Care needs to be taken that the chart of accounts does not become too cumbersome with unneeded items. The example in Figure 8-12 details all of the costs related to telephone and pager services that can be charged to a single line item or broken down into more specific line items.

SALARIES & BENEFITS:
Salaries & Draws: Owner
Salaries & Wages: Full-Time
Salaries & Wages: Part-Time
Overtime
Health Insurance: Owner
Health Insurance: Staff
Retirement Plan: Owner
Retirement Plan: Staff
Other Benefits

OPERATING EXPENSES:
Office Supplies
Patient Care Supplies
Insurance: Malpractice
Insurance: Other
Accounting & Legal
Advertising
Travel & Training
Memberships & Subscriptions
Meals & Meetings
Postage
Donations
Repairs & Maintenance
Licenses & Taxes
Uniforms & Cleaning
Telephone & Pagers
Utilities

CAPITAL & DEBT
Lease Payments: Office
Lease Payments: Equipment
Principal on Loans
Interest on Loans
Equipment
Land & Buildings

© Cengage Learning 2013

Figure 8-11 Chart of accounts listing specific line items that are tracked in the budget.

2150	Telephone & Pagers	7,500
	OR	
2151	Telephone Service	3,600
2152	Answering Service	2,400
2153	Cell Phones & Pagers	1,500

© Cengage Learning 2013

Figure 8-12 Account Detail of how Costs are Charged to Line Items

The revenue budget for the practice is prepared in the same manner. A chart of accounts for revenues is developed, setting individual line revenue line items for each source of revenue. Revenues will include fees for medical service from private-pay patients, insurance reimbursements, and government payments from programs such as Medicare and Medicaid.

Step Two: Track Historical Revenues and Costs

The budget for the next year cannot be accurately completed without knowing how much has been spent in prior years and how much is expected to be spent in the current year. The accounting system used by the practice should be able to provide detailed expenditures in prior years that can be placed into the appropriate categories in the chart of accounts. Expenditures for the current year are projected using prior years' actual costs, taking into account inflation and any changes in the medical practice that will impact costs. Statistical reports result from 1 year of operations in an organization. This year then becomes a prior year report and is part of the history of the organization. Most organizations do historical budgeting, so the finance department and the nurse manager refer to prior year reports when creating the budget for the next fiscal year.

Revenues from prior years will be recorded and current year revenues will be projected.

Step Three: Benchmark Costs

Salaries that are too low or benefits below those normally offered in the area will result in poor morale and high staff turnover. Salaries and benefits that are too high can seriously impact the financial health of the practice. Too few staff will hurt the effective delivery of medical services, and too large a staff is financially wasteful. Bench marking, addressed earlier, is designed to staff the facility with the appropriate number of employees for each function. One of the responsibilities of the human resources department is to ensure that salaries and benefits are competitive in the local market area.

Step Four: Build the Annual Budget

The annual budget is based on where the practice has been and any changes that are expected for the upcoming budget year. Any proposed changes in fees charged to private-pay patients and reimbursement rates from insurance companies need to be considered. Economic changes in the community, such as a factory closing or a new business coming to town, will affect patient load. The physician and practice manager will meet to discuss these issues as well as staffing levels and proposed pay changes for the upcoming year. Using historical data from prior years and the current year for each individual line item, and making adjustments for changes in costs, each line item is budgeted for the upcoming year. The total of the expenditure budget is then compared to projected revenues for the year to ensure that the plan is financially feasible. An example of an industry trend is a change in technology. For example, some orthopedic total hip replacements now take an anterior approach, with the patient discharged the next day rather than enduring a 3-day hospital stay. This affects reimbursement. Another example is the use of percutaneous cardiac interventions rather than coronary bypass surgery in myocardial infarction patients. Other industry trends could relate to things happening in politics, such as decreasing reimbursement in the Medicare or Medicaid programs.

Step Five: Review the Monthly Budget

To serve as an effective tool for the management of the practice, actual expenses for each month need to be compared to the annual budget. Not all expenses will be paid in equal monthly installments. Some costs, such as insurance premiums, may be paid monthly, quarterly, semiannually, or even annually. The timing of these expenses needs to be taken into consideration when reviewing the actual expenses against the budget to ensure that the practice is operating within the budget. The practice manager should do a thorough review of each month's expenses and plan to spend a few minutes with the physician to review any important issues arising from the review. One of the highest costs of inventory in a hospital is the operating room. In most operating rooms, surgeons have a procedure card for each type of surgical procedure that the respective surgeon performs. The procedure cards list all the items or inventory required for the procedure.

Any significant issues raised through this process of variance analysis should be resolved immediately before they become a serious problem.

Knowledge Check 8.5

1. Explain the steps involved in developing an effective budget for a smaller medical facility.

_____

_____

_____

2. What is the purpose of a monthly review of actual experience against the annual budget of the facility?

_____

_____

_____

Break-Even Analysis

A fundamental question in budgeting for healthcare organizations is, "How many patients (or clients) do we need to see to cover our costs for the year?" The concept of **break-even analysis** provides a mechanism to answer this question. To determine the break-even point, the **fixed costs** are first calculated. Fixed costs are those costs that will be incurred before the first patient is seen. These costs will include salaries and benefits of the permanent staff, depreciation of capital assets, and administrative overhead. **Variable costs** are expenses of doing business that are based on the number of units of service provided. Variable costs will include medical and operating supplies, lab tests, and housekeeping costs. The number of units of service required to cover both the fixed and variable costs is determined by the following equation:

$$\text{Price} \times \text{Volume} = \text{Fixed Costs} + (\text{Variable Cost per Unit} \times \text{Volume})$$

Example 8-3

Sunnydale Home Health Services is a small company, meeting the home care needs of residents of the local community. Sunnydale has a staff of two registered nurses and two nursing assistants. Total fixed costs, including staff salaries and benefits, has been calculated at $250,000 annually. Indirect costs, including supplies and the cost of vehicle use, has been identified at $25 per unit of service. The average revenue for each unit of service is $75. Using the previous break-even equation, the break-even point is calculated as:

$$\$75 \times \text{Volume} = \$250,000 + (\$25 \times \text{Volume})$$

Volume, the total number of units of service that need to be provided for Sunnydale to break even for the year, is thus 5,000. Each unit of service provides $50 ($75 per unit revenue less $25 variable cost) toward fixed costs. Thus, $250,000 total fixed costs divided by $50 equals the 5,000 units of service required.

Figure 8-13 shows the break-even point of patients that need to be seen for a healthcare facility to make a profit. This is determined by the following equation:

Patient Visits = Fixed Costs/Revenue Per Visit − Variable Costs

If the healthcare facility is losing money, there are several options to improve the outcome.

1. Renegotiate with the payers for higher rates. Conduct market research to see if the institution is charging below the market rate.

2. Look for ways to increase patient traffic. Accept new patients, send out appointment reminders, and consider extending hours.

3. Reduce fixed costs.

4. Look for ways to reduce your variable costs, too. This may mean staff reductions, outsourcing, cheaper alternatives or substitutes for goods or services, or switching vendors.

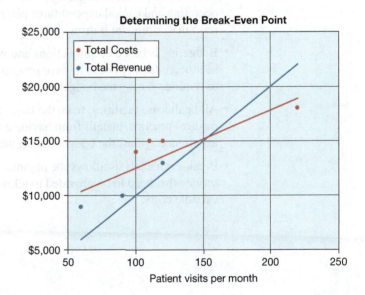

Figure 8-13 Patient Visits

Key Concepts

- The budget represents management's plan, expressed in dollars, for a future period of time.

- Annual operating budgets are prepared for each work unit in the healthcare facility and combined into a master operating budget.

- In addition to operating budgets that provide detail on annual expenditures, authorized personnel budgets detail the number of personnel positions approved, the capital budget itemizes the replacement of worn-out or obsolete capital equipment over a period of several years, the statistical and revenue budgets project revenues for the facility, and the cash budget describes the cash flow impact of monthly changes to revenues and expenditures during the budget year.

- In top-down budgeting, senior management and finance staff control the budget development process. In bottom-up budgeting, individual unit managers are heavily involved in the final determination of their unit's budgets.

- Incremental budgeting starts with the current year's approved budget and adds funds to account for inflation and workload changes. In zero-base budgeting, every position authorized and the budget for each line item must be justified from a base of zero.

- The final step in the budgeting process is balancing the budget to ensure that the operating and capital expenditures planned for the budget year will be supported by revenues or prudent borrowing.

- Budgeting is based on projections and will never be completely accurate. Each healthcare facility needs to have programs in place to control and amend the budget as required during the budget year.

- All healthcare facilities, from the largest hospital to the smallest single-physician medical practice, benefit from having a budget and continuously monitoring actual experience against the budget during the year.

- Break-even analysis allows the organization to calculate the number of units of service that need to be provided to allow the organization to cover both fixed and variable costs.

Cash Management

Key Terms

Bank reconciliation
Cash and cash equivalents
Cash drawer
Float
Petty cash fund
Stale-dated checks
Statement of cash flows

Chapter Objectives

After completing this chapter, readers should be able to:

- Identify the basic cash management tools used by any medical facility, including the petty cash fund, the cash drawer, and the operating checking account.

- Demonstrate the ability to properly prepare a bank reconciliation.

- Describe the development and use of the statement of cash flows.

- Illustrate the importance of cash management in ensuring adequate cash resources to operate the business.

Chapter Glossary

Bank reconciliation is the process of ensuring that the accounting records for the checking account agree with the monthly bank statement.

Cash and cash equivalents on the balance sheet combines cash, checking account balances, and short-term liquid investments such as certificates of deposit or treasury bills.

The **cash drawer**, generally part of a cash register linked to the financial management system, is used to make change for patients paying cash for services provided.

Float refers to the length of time from the date a check is written until the check clears the issuing bank and funds are withdrawn from the issuer's account.

The **petty cash fund** of a business is used to account for small cash expenditures.

Stale-dated checks are checks issued by a business that have not been presented for payment within a reasonable period of time.

The **statement of cash flows** supplements the balance sheet and income statement, providing the reader with information on the sources and uses of cash in the business.

Introduction

Cash management is a process that includes all personnel of the organization involved with the business side of the operation. In a small medical office, this will include the practice manager and any staff in the accounting, cashiering, and billing functions. In a larger facility, such as a hospital, this will include all of the personnel assigned finance and accounting responsibilities. The process involves accurate cash handling, daily bank deposits, accurate and timely billing to third-party payers such as Medicare and insurance companies, investment of cash not needed immediately for operating needs, bank reconciliations, and monitoring of cash flow. Appropriate financial controls are built into the system and continually monitored by supervisory personnel. Modern financial management technology provides significant assistance in cash management; however, technology does not replace trained and dedicated employees.

Cash Management Tools

Cash management for any business starts with the basics: a petty cash fund, a cash drawer to handle daily cash received as payment for goods or services, and a business checking account to account for both cash received into the business and cash distributions to pay the costs of running the business.

Petty Cash

The widespread use of both credit and debit cards for business has reduced, but not eliminated, the use of a **petty cash fund** for business. The petty cash fund is used to reimburse employees of the business for miscellaneous purchases. These routine business expenses are best accounted for with a petty cash fund. A physician uses their own cash to attend a meeting in the city. A business document has additional postage due. An employee of the medical practice buys doughnuts for a morning staff meeting. In each of these examples, use of petty cash is more appropriate than writing a business check for the expense.

A petty cash fund gives a small business the flexibility of quickly reimbursing or paying small expenditures without having to write a company check or use a company credit card. An employee can run out to the post office, not knowing the exact amount of postage needed on an item for the mail, taking petty cash with them to pay for the expenditure.

Companies typically keep between $30 and $300 in their petty cash funds. The use of petty cash is only appropriate for small, erratic expenses that pop up unexpectedly.

Case Study 9-1

Dr. Powers operates a single-provider family medical practice. One medical assistant handles appointments, basic bookkeeping functions, and assists with medical records. Two additional medical assistants assist in patient care. The physician's spouse comes into the office on an irregular basis to prepare the bank deposit. The accountant for the practice has been able to convince Dr. Powers to hire a practice manager, rather than another medical assistant, to manage the increasing workload of the practice.

Teresa Ruiz has been hired into the position of practice manager and has arrived for her first day of work. The medical assistant responsible for opening the mail and posting patient payments tells Ms. Ruiz that patient records are up to date on payments received and charges for services, but she has been instructed to only place the cash and checks received into the cash drawer and that Dr. Powers' spouse would handle the cash from that point. In the cash drawer, Ms. Ruiz finds checks dated over the past 2 weeks, cash far in excess of that needed for daily operations, and dozens of IOUs where Dr. Powers has taken cash from the cash drawer for lunches.

What are the appropriate steps for Ms. Ruiz to take to establish reasonable financial controls over the cash handling process?

A petty cash fund is first established by writing a check for the amount of the initial deposit to the fund. The amount of the fund should be sufficient to meet expenses for a reasonable period of time before the fund needs to be replenished, but not excessive where theft becomes a temptation. The initial deposit to the fund is not an expense, so the offset to the credit in the checking account cash balance will be the creation of an asset account called petty cash.

The petty cash custodian has purchased a locking cash box and a pad of petty cash expense forms from the local office supply store. The petty cash fund is now open for business. An employee uses their own money for an approved business expense. They obtain a receipt from the vendor and present the receipt to the petty cash custodian. The employee is reimbursed for the expense from the fund, the expense form is completed, and the vendor receipt is stapled to the expense form. As other transactions are completed, the petty cash fund begins to run low on cash. The custodian requests a check from accounting made out to cash in the amount of the total of the expense forms provided with the check request. The custodian cashes the check at their bank, and the fund is replenished to the original amount. The petty cash fund will always be replenished to the original amount at the end of each fiscal year so that the accounting records properly reflect both the account balance and expenses incurred that year.

Even though petty cash is designed to be a minor part of cash management, financial controls need to be in place. One individual is charged with the responsibility of petty cash custodian and is held accountable for the accuracy of the fund. Receipts are required for all reimbursements and all expenditures are approved in advance. Petty cash reimbursements are always made through the petty cash fund, never through the cash drawer. The petty cash custodian should not be the individual who prepares the check for replenishing the fund. These simple controls will protect the fund from abuse.

The Cash Drawer and the Cash Receipts Process

The **cash drawer** is used to account for payments made by customers during the course of the business day and to make change for customers. Cash in this context includes coins, paper money, and checks that are received, either in person or by mail, in payment for services provided. The beginning balance in the cash drawer will be based on the volume of cash transactions made during the day. In a medical practice where most patients pay by credit card, a small cash balance, say $100, may be sufficient. Cash will be broken down into denominations appropriate to make change for patients.

Because cash can easily be lost, proper internal controls must be established over the cash handling process. The simplest of these is separation of responsibilities in the process of receiving cash, making change for the patient from the cash drawer, and preparing the bank deposit. One employee should be responsible for accepting cash payments from patients and daily balancing of the cash drawer. Once the daily balancing has been completed and the bank deposit prepared, the cash drawer should have the same balance as at the start of the day. All patients should be provided with a receipt for payments made. When the receipt is computer generated, the entry in the computer will correspond to the cash received into the cash drawer.

For payments received by mail, one employee opens the mail and stamps the back of each check with a secured endorsement, showing the name of the facility, the bank account number, and the mark "For Deposit Only." A second employee makes the computer entries to record the payments to the patient's account.

A third employee reconciles the bank deposit to the computer-generated daily cash receipts journal and makes the bank deposit. This separation of responsibilities works well in larger medical offices and hospitals that have a large enough office staff to provide for the separation of duties. Smaller medical offices need to understand the risks involved in having one employee in charge of the full cycle of cash receipts and take steps that are reasonable to provide oversight.

Cash Disbursements

Payments made by the medical office to pay for the various costs of doing business require their own set of controls. Some vendors will provide a discount for prompt payments, and the accounting system should be structured to take advantage of these discounts when offered. Vendors will also commonly charge a penalty for late payment as an incentive to pay invoices when due. In a small medical office, the physician may sign the checks or may delegate the responsibility to the practice manager. In either case, the person signing the checks will most likely have a good understanding of the size and frequency of the costs of running the business and will be able to spot any questionable payments. In larger facilities, internal control procedures are established to ensure that all payments made are appropriate. These internal control procedures will include detailed requirements prior to payment of any invoices by accounting: each request for payment includes a vendor invoice, purchase order, and delivery ticket signed to indicate receipt of the proper materials in good condition. A payment voucher is prepared and signed by a supervisor, indicating the proper account code to be charged for the expenditure. Control procedures over cash disbursements are also established within the accounting department. Payments are made on a periodic basis, generally once a week. Checks are cut by the staff in the accounting department and, prior to mailing, are reviewed by an accounting supervisor. The accounting supervisor reviews both the checks and the documentation for each payment and reviews the payments to the weekly edit listing of payments. A check log is prepared to ensure that there are no unexplained breaks in check number sequence. The accounting supervisor initials both the weekly check edit listing and the check log. Blank checks are properly secured.

Comprehension Check 9.1

1. The office manager of an outpatient facility is responsible for reimbursing employees of the business for miscellaneous purchases. Which cash management tool is being used?

2. Dr. Bernu wants to save time on accounting needs for the practice. Since this one factor is the largest in the practice, the decision was made to outsource this to a service provider. Which cash management tool is being used?

3. Senior medical assistant Hannah is responsible for making change for all the cash paying patients at Quonto Diagnostic Center. Which cash management tool is being used?

Businesses are not limited to a single checking account. As facilities grow, many find it advantageous to maintain separate accounts for specific purposes. Commonly, a medical facility will maintain a separate checking account for payroll. Payments to employees represent the largest single cost factor for a medical facility, and a separate account provides for greater accountability of these expenditures. Due to the complexity of payroll and the requirement that payroll is both accurate and timely, many medical facilities have chosen to outsource the responsibility to a service provider. In many cases, the costs of the payroll service company will prove to be less than the costs of preparing payroll in-house, freeing up the time of employees to accomplish other accounting tasks. In either case, the payroll checking account is maintained with a zero balance, and the amount of the payroll transferred from the operating checking account into the payroll checking account as the periodic payroll is issued.

Knowledge Check 9.1

1. Mrs. Ivanov comes into the medical facility for a routine office visit. Her copayment is $35, and she hands the cashier a $50 bill. The $50 bill is deposited into, and the $15 change is taken from, which of the following?
   A. Petty cash fund
   B. Cash drawer
   C. Operating checking account
   D. Payroll checking account

2. Johnson's Carpet Cleaning has completed their monthly cleaning at the medical office and submitted their billing for $200. Payment to Johnson's is made from the:
   A. Petty cash fund
   B. Cash drawer
   C. Operating checking account
   D. Payroll checking account

3. Drs. Sawyer and Preston operate a medical partnership. An employee has been designated and trained as a cashier, responsible for opening the mail and recording payments received. The cashier also takes payments from patients receiving medical services. The cashier balances the cash

continued

drawer, prepares the daily bank deposit, and drops the deposit into the bank's night deposit at the end of the day. What recommendations would you make to improve internal controls over the cash handling process?

_____

_____

_____

4. Mr. Alvarez has just been named as the practice manager for a three-doctor urology practice. Mr. Alvarez is reviewing the petty cash fund and notices that there are several hundred dollars in cash as well as IOUs from various employees in the fund. Dr. Singh, the senior partner, tells Mr. Alvarez that the practice allows employees to use cash from the petty cash fund to tide them over until payday. What do you think of this policy?

_____

_____

_____

5. In the case study at the beginning of the chapter, Ms. Ruiz has just been hired as practice manager and has concerns about how cash is handled by the practice. What changes should Ms. Ruiz make to Dr. Powers' practice?

_____

_____

_____

Bank Reconciliation

Banks will provide their business customers with a monthly statement of activity on each checking account. The balance on the bank statement as of the cutoff date will not equal the accounting ledger balance for that same account as of that same date. There are two primary reasons for this difference: (1) timing issues of the uncleared deposits made and checks issued by the medical facility, and (2) bank adjustments for interest paid on the account and for bank charges to the account. Balancing the bank statement to the ledger balance for cash in the account is called **bank reconciliation**. See Figure 9-1 for an example of a blank bank reconciliation statement.

Bank reconciliation is a three-step process:

Step 1: Mark all deposits in the facility's accounting records that agree to deposits on the bank statement. Also mark as cleared all checks issued that appear as paid on the bank statement. All deposits and checks written that are not marked as in agreement between the accounting records and the bank statement are items that did not clear the bank as of the statement date and will need to be shown on the reconciliation.

Step 2: Adjust the bank statement for all items that did not clear the bank as of the statement date. The most common variance for deposits will be the deposit by the medical facility made late in the day of the statement date. The deposit was entered for that date by the medical facility but will appear on the bank statement as of the next business date. Most likely, there will be numerous checks written by the medical facility that are outstanding as of the bank statement date. A check is prepared and mailed by the facility near the bank statement date. By the time the mail reaches the vendor, the vendor deposits

Morningside Medical Clinic
Bank Reconciliation
DATE:

Balance per Bank Statement _____

ADD: Deposits in Transit:

DATE	AMOUNT

_____

LESS: Checks Outstanding:

CHECK#	AMOUNT		CHECK#	AMOUNT

Adjusted Bank Balance ===========

Cash Balance per Accounting Records _____

ADD: Interest Received   [JOURNAL ENTRY]   _____

LESS: Bank Charges   [JOURNAL ENTRY]   _____

LESS: Credit Card Fees   [JOURNAL ENTRY]   _____

LESS: Non-Sufficient Funds Checks   [JOURNAL ENTRY]   _____

Other Reconciling Items   [JOURNAL ENTRY]   _____

Adjusted Cash Balance ===========

Figure 9-1 A Blank Example of a Bank Reconciliation Statement

the check in their bank, and the bank forwards the check to the facility's bank for payment, a number of days have passed and the check has not cleared by the date of the bank statement. This delay, between the date that the check is issued and the date when the check clears the issuing bank, is referred to as **float**. During this float period, the issuer has the use of the funds and, when using a checking account with interest, will be earning interest on the funds. Each of the checks issued that have not cleared the bank by the statement date will need to be listed and the total of outstanding checks used as a reconciling item.

Checks that have not cleared the bank for a lengthy period of time are referred to as **stale-dated checks**. Periodically, these stale-dated checks need to be removed from the accounting records. The process involves contacting the check payee to determine the status of the check. If the check has been lost in the mail or misplaced by the payee, the original check will be voided, the check reissued, and a stop-payment order on the original check sent to the bank. When the payee cannot be found, perhaps issued to a company no longer in business, state law will govern the disposition of the funds. In many states, the check will be voided, a stop-payment order sent to the bank, and the funds deposited with the state's unclaimed property office.

Step 3: Identify those items on the bank statement that will need to be recorded in the financial records of the medical facility. In Figure 9-1, these items are identified where the shaded box says JOURNAL ENTRY. Items that will require a journal entry are recorded on the bank reconciliation form, and a journal entry is prepared and entered into the financial records. These items will include interest paid by the bank on the account, bank charges for the month, fees for payments made with the patient's credit card, any checks that have not cleared the bank due to non-sufficient funds (NSF checks), and any other reconciling items that appear on the bank statement. When the bank statement includes an NSF check, the individual patient account will need to be adjusted to remove the payment and any fee charged for NSF checks added to the amount due on the patient account. Journal entries to record interest earned and bank charges would be prepared as shown in Figure 9-2.

JOURNAL ENTRY

ACCOUNT NUMBER	DESCRIPTION	DEBIT	CREDIT
	Cash—Operating Checking	12.00	
	Interest Earned		12.00
	Bank Charges	25.00	
	Cash—Operating Checking		25.00

Figure 9-2 Journal Entries Recording Earned Interest and Bank Charges

These two journal entries in Figure 9-2 may also be combined into a single entry as demonstrated in Figure 9-3.

JOURNAL ENTRY

ACCOUNT NUMBER	DESCRIPTION	DEBIT	CREDIT
	Cash—Operating Checking		13.00
	Interest Earned		12.00
	Bank Charges	25.00	

Figure 9-3 A Single Journal Entry Recording Earned Interest and Bank Charges

Bank reconciliation becomes more complicated when dealing with automated payment processes. A patient is provided with medical services and pays the $35 office visit copayment by credit card. The medical facility forwards the credit card payment to the credit card company for payment. When the payment is received by the bank, the amount paid by the credit card company will be shown as the full amount of the charge, in this case $35, with the service charge from the credit card company shown separately. The balance of the fee for the office visit is submitted to the group health insurance plan covering the patient. Payment will be deposited directly into the operating bank account of the facility with an itemized report sent directly to the facility. In a busy medical practice or in a hospital, these direct payments into the bank and reports to the facility will be a daily occurrence. Frequently, the combination of the copayment received from the patient and the payment from the insurance company will not equal the standard charge for service of the medical facility. In these cases, the remaining balance will be written off. Chapter 7 included a discussion on the proper accounting treatment in cases where the combination of patient responsibility and payment from a third-party payer is less than the amount originally recorded as revenues from a medical procedure.

A completed bank reconciliation is shown in Figure 9-4.

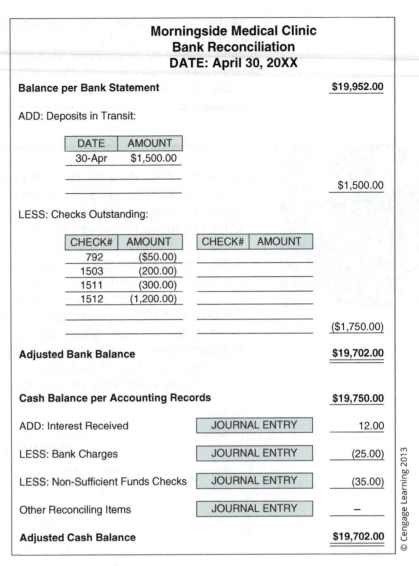

Figure 9-4 A Completed Bank Reconciliation Form for Morningside
Medical Clinic

The adjusted cash balance, in this example $19,702.00, is compared to the cash balance in the accounting records after the journal entry has been entered. If the adjusted cash balance per the bank reconciliation agrees to the cash balance in the accounting records, the reconciliation is complete. If the two numbers do not agree, there is an error that needs to be found and corrected. There could be an error in the facility's accounting records or the error could have been caused by the bank. The easiest error to detect would be one made during the reconciliation process. Double-check the mathematical accuracy of the bank reconciliation form, or if using a spreadsheet, verify that the formulas are accurate. Double-check all entries on the bank reconciliation form to ensure the accuracy of the entries. Any omissions on month-end deposits in transit or outstanding checks will cause the reconciliation to be in error. Double-check each of the items on the reconciliation that require a journal entry. Verify that each item from the bank statement is present on the reconciliation, that each is correct as to an addition to or subtraction from the bank statement balance, and that the journal entry posted agrees with the bank reconciliation. If these actions do not uncover the variance, a detailed review of each item for the month in both the facility's accounting records and in the bank statement will need to be started. Both the accounting records and the bank statement are simply lists of numbers, and one pair of these numbers does not match.

Modern computer software has made the process of bank reconciliation much easier. What used to be a manual process using a pencil to mark off items and an adding machine to prove the final balance has been replaced with computer files downloaded from the bank. Smaller medical offices will use computer programs for cash management that allow bank reconciliation through a simple process of responding to prompts in the program.

Knowledge Check 9.2

1. At the statement date, the bank shows a balance in the facility's operating checking account of $10,000. On that same statement date, the facility's accounting records have a cash balance in the operating account of $10,525 and has recorded a deposit of $1,000 that the bank does not show. Also, the facility has issued three checks, in the amounts of $100, $200, and $300, that the bank does not show as cleared. For that month, the bank has credited interest to the account in the amount of $25 and has charged bank service fees of $50. Credit card service fees for the month total $100. All payments from third-party payers on the bank statement agree to the facility's accounting records. Prepare the journal entry to record interest and charges, and complete the bank reconciliation to determine the adjusted cash balance per the facility's accounting records.
   A blank bank reconciliation form for your use is on the following page.

JOURNAL ENTRY			
ACCOUNT NUMBER	**DESCRIPTION**	**DEBIT**	**CREDIT**

© Cengage Learning 2013

2. Working in a single-physician medical office, Aaron Hoffman serves as cashier for the office, makes the daily bank deposit, and is responsible for the monthly bank reconciliation. What recommendations would you make to improve internal control in this area?

_____

_____

_____

3. The accountant for a community hospital is preparing the monthly bank reconciliation and notices that a large check issued for medical supplies has been outstanding for more than 6 months. What are the appropriate steps that should be taken with this stale-dated check?

_____

_____

_____

continued

Bank Reconciliation
DATE:

Balance per Bank Statement _____

ADD: Deposits in Transit:

DATE	AMOUNT

_____

LESS: Checks Outstanding:

CHECK#	AMOUNT	CHECK#	AMOUNT

Adjusted Bank Balance _____

Cash Balance per Accounting Records _____

ADD: Interest Received | JOURNAL ENTRY | _____

LESS: Bank Charges | JOURNAL ENTRY | _____

LESS: Credit Card Fees | JOURNAL ENTRY | _____

LESS: Non-Sufficient Funds Checks | JOURNAL ENTRY | _____

Other Reconciling Items | JOURNAL ENTRY | _____

Adjusted Cash Balance _____

The Statement of Cash Flows

The **statement of cash flows** is a fairly recent addition to generally accepted accounting principles (GAAP). The statement of cash flows is now a required third statement, supplementing the information in the balance sheet and income statement. The statement serves as a means to make the conversion from accrual accounting to cash accounting, reporting on where the business generates cash and what the cash is used for. Cash flow is divided into three sections, as shown in Figure 9-5.

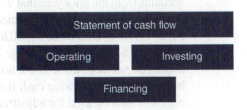

Figure 9-5 Statement of Cash Flow

Cash management, like everything else in the business world, begins with reliable information. The two primary business reports, discussed in previous chapters, are the balance sheet and the income statement. The balance sheet provides a snapshot of the financial position of the business at a certain point in time, and the income statement provides details on revenues and expenses over a period of time. An income statement will always be prepared annually for the fiscal year of the medical facility but may also be prepared on a monthly or quarterly basis depending on the needs of management. A third statement becomes necessary in order to manage the cash of the organization: the statement of cash flows. The balance sheet will show the cash position of the business at a single date in time but will provide no information as to how cash is generated by business activities. The income statement will show the net operating income for a period of time but lacks the correlation between net income and cash available to continue to operate the business.

The concept of accrual accounting becomes critically important in the consideration of cash flows. Revenues and cash availability do not occur on the same date except when a patient makes a cash payment at time of service. Payments made by credit card take a number of days to become cash when funds are received from the credit card company. There is an even longer time lag when patients or third-party payers need to be billed for services provided.

Example 9-1

The Morningside Medical Clinic operates on a December 31 fiscal year. Patients are seen throughout the month of December, but payments from insurance are not made until January, the following fiscal year. If Morningside operated on a cash basis, no revenues other than deductibles and copayments would be recorded as revenues for December. Under accrual accounting, patient charges during December are posted as revenues and the offsetting entries are a combination of cash received from patients and accounts receivable.

On the expense side, Morningside purchases supplies, uses utilities, and charges services from outside vendors in December as in any other month. These operating expenses are not paid until January; however, under accrual accounting, the costs are charged to December activity with the offsetting entry of accounts payable. These revenues and expenses will be included in Morningside's income statement for the year ending December 31, but the cash account will not be affected until revenues are received and bills paid in January. The statement of cash flows will make the necessary adjustments to operating net income to reflect the actual impact on cash flow.

The statement of cash flows for Morningside for 2020, with comparative data for 2019, is shown in Figure 9-6.

The statement of cash flows for Morningside starts with net income taken directly from the income statement. The first step in the conversion from net income to cash flows is to make adjustments for any non-cash items that affect net income. The most common of these is the annual charge for depreciation, the periodic writing down of the value of long-term assets owned by the business. Depreciation is taken directly from the income statement and added back to net income.

Following the adjustment for depreciation are changes in any asset and liability accounts from the prior year that will affect net income and cash flow. Assume as an example that Morningside had a balance in accounts receivable of $200,000 as of December 31, 2019. As of December 31, 2020, the accounts receivable balance has increased to the amount of $227,000. This change in the year-end balance of accounts receivable has no impact on net income for 2020; however, the increase in the accounts receivable balance has resulted in decreasing cash flow for 2020 in the amount of $27,000. This same process will then be used for adjustments to other current asset accounts such as inventory and prepaid expenses and for current liability accounts such as accounts payable. The

Morningside Medical Clinic
Statement of Cash Flows
For the Year Ending December 31, 2020
(With Comparative Data for 2019)

	December 31, 2020	December 31, 2019
Operating Net Income	$146,500	$97,250
Reconciliation of Net Income to Cash Flow:		
Add Back: Depreciation and Amortization	35,000	35,000
(Increase)/Decrease in Accounts Receivable	(27,000)	22,500
(Increase)/Decrease in Inventory	2,000	(1,000)
(Increase)/Decrease in Prepaid Expenses	2,500	1,500
Increase/(Decrease) in Accounts Payable	5,000	2,000
Adjustments to Net Income	17,500	60,000
NET CASH FLOW FROM OPERATIONS	**$164,000**	**$157,250**
CASH & CASH EQUIVALENTS, BEGINNING OF YEAR	239,250	82,000
CASH & CASH EQUIVALENTS, END OF YEAR	**$403,250**	**$239,250**

Figure 9-6 Morningside Medical Clinic Cash Flow Statement with Comparative Data for Present Year and Year Prior

total amount of these adjustments will then be added to or subtracted from net income to determine net cash flow from operations. The net cash flow from operations reflects the actual annual impact on cash from the operations of the business for the year.

Cash and cash equivalents are the combined total of the balances in cash accounts such as petty cash and operating checking accounts and cash equivalents, defined as financial assets such as money market accounts or short-term investments that may be converted to cash. Figure 9-7 shows some examples of cash and cash equivalents.

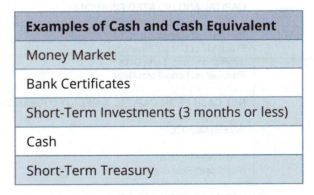

Examples of Cash and Cash Equivalent
Money Market
Bank Certificates
Short-Term Investments (3 months or less)
Cash
Short-Term Treasury

Figure 9-7 Examples of Cash and Cash Equivalents

The proof of the accuracy of the statement of cash flows is shown at the bottom of the analysis. For any fiscal year, cash and cash equivalents at the end of the prior fiscal year become the beginning balance in cash and cash equivalents for the new fiscal year. Adding the net cash flow from operations to the beginning balance of cash and cash equivalents yields the balance in cash and cash equivalents at the end of the fiscal year. This number is then tied back to the balance sheet amount for cash and cash equivalents to determine accuracy.

Figure 9-8 determines the net cash flow from operations. To complete the statement of cash flows, further adjustments need to be made if the business purchased any capital assets during the year, with or without outside financing, or had purchased or sold investments that are not accounted for in cash and cash equivalents. Near the end of 2009, Morningside purchased a piece of medical equipment at a cost of $150,000, financing $120,000 with the equipment manufacturer over 6 years at an annual interest rate of 6 percent. During 2010, Morningside made the first payments of interest and principal on this debt. Morningside also has a policy of investing cash not needed immediately for the operation of the business in bank certificates of deposit maturing in 1 to 2 years. The statement of cash flows will then also include a section showing the impact on cash flows from both interest earned on investments and the purchase or sale of investments. The statement of cash flows now includes three separate sections detailing the impact on cash flows: net cash from operations, net cash from capital and related financing, and net cash from operations.

Morningside Medical Clinic
Statement of Cash Flows
For the Year Ending December 31, 2020
(With Comparative Data for 2019)

	December 31, 2020	December 31, 2019
Operating Net Income	$146,500	$97,250
Reconciliation of Net Income to Cash Flow:		
Add Back: Depreciation and Amortization	35,000	35,000
(Increase)/Decrease in Accounts Receivable	(27,000)	22,500
(Increase)/Decrease in Inventory	2,000	(1,000)
(Increase)/Decrease in Prepaid Expenses	2,500	1,500
Increase/(Decrease) in Accounts Payable	5,000	2,000
Adjustments to Net Income	17,500	60,000
NET CASH FLOW FROM OPERATIONS	164,000	157,250
CAPITAL AND RELATED FINANCING:		
Purchase of Capital Equipment	–	(150,000)
Proceeds of Capital Financing	–	120,000
Interest on Long-Term Debt	(7,200)	–
Principal on Long-Term Debt	(20,000)	–
NET CASH FROM CAPITAL & RELATED FINANCING	(27,200)	(30,000)
INVESTMENTS:		
Investment Income	6,500	2,000
(Purchase)/Sale of Investments	(250,000)	(50,000)
NET CASH FROM INVESTMENTS	(243,500)	(30,000)
NET INCREASE IN CASH & CASH EQUIVALENTS	($106,700)	$97,250
CASH & CASH EQUIVALENTS, BEGINNING OF YEAR	179,250	82,000
CASH & CASH EQUIVALENTS, END OF YEAR	$72,550	$179,250

© Cengage Learning 2013

Figure 9-8 Completed Cash Flow Statement for Morningside Medical Clinic

Comprehension Check 9.2

1. Centra Medical Center is reviewing the statement of cash flows. By reviewing the cash flow operating costs, cash flow investing costs, and cash flow financing costs, what would be the net increase in cash and cash equivalents?

Centra Medical Center Statement of Cash Flows Year Ended xxx - Indicates decrease in cash	
Cash Flow Operating Costs	
Supplies	-$10,000
Rent	-$30,000
Security Deposit	-$5,000
Total Cash Flow from Operations	-$45,000
Cash Flow from Investing	
Medical Equipment	-$10,000
Purchase of Computers	-$20,000
Purchase of Billing Software	-$5,000
Total Cash Flow from Investing	-$35,000
Cash Flow from Financing	
Owners Investment	$198,000
Total Cash Flow from Financing	$198,000
Net Increase in Cash and Cash Equivalents	

Knowledge Check

9.3

1. All of the following would be included in cash and cash equivalents EXCEPT:

A. Petty cash fund

B. Cash drawer

C. Operating checking account

D. Bank certificates of deposit that mature in 2 years

2. On the following form, complete the statement of cash flows for the year ending December 31, 2020, to determine cash flow from operations and changes in cash and cash equivalents, using the following data: 2020 depreciation was $20,000, accounts receivable were down by $10,000 from 12/31/19, and inventory, prepaid expenses, and accounts payable balances all increased by $1,000 from the prior year-end:

Statement of Cash Flows
For the Year Ending December 31, 2020
(With Comparative Data for 2019)

	December 31, 2020	December 31, 2019
Operating Net Income	$110,000	$100,000
Reconciliation of Net Income to Cash Flow:		
Add Back: Depreciation and Amortization		20,000
(Increase)/Decrease in Accounts Receivable		10,000
(Increase)/Decrease in Inventory		(1,000)
(Increase)/Decrease in Prepaid Expenses		1,500
Increase/(Decrease) in Accounts Payable	_____	2,000
Adjustments to Net Income		32,500
NET CASH FLOW FROM OPERATIONS	══════	$132,500
CASH & CASH EQUIVALENTS, BEGINNING OF YEAR		50,000
CASH & CASH EQUIVALENTS, END OF YEAR	══════	$182,500

continued

3. Beginning with cash flow from operations calculated in question 2, complete the following statement of cash flows, using the following additional information: During 2020, the facility purchased a piece of capital equipment for cash for $50,000, interest on long-term debt was $5,000, and principal on long-term debt was $10,000. During the year, $100,000 in available cash was used to purchase an investment. Investment income for the year was $3,000.

Statement of Cash Flows
For the Year Ending December 31, 2020
(With Comparative Data for 2019)

	December 31, 2020	December 31, 2019
Operating Net Income	$110,000	$100,000
Reconciliation of Net Income to Cash Flow:		
Add Back: Depreciation and Amortization		20,000
(Increase)/Decrease in Accounts Receivable		10,000
(Increase)/Decrease in Inventory		(1,000)
(Increase)/Decrease in Prepaid Expenses		1,500
Increase/(Decrease) in Accounts Payable	_____	2,000
Adjustments to Net Income		32,500
NET CASH FLOW FROM OPERATIONS		132,500
CAPITAL AND RELATED FINANCING:		
Purchase of Capital Equipment		—
Proceeds of Capital Financing		—
Interest on Long-Term Debt		(5,000)
Principal on Long-Term Debt		(10,000)
NET CASH FROM CAPITAL & RELATED FINANCING	—	(15,000)
INVESTMENTS:		
Investment Income		3,000
(Purchase)/Sale of Investments		—
NET CASH FROM INVESTMENTS	_____	2,000
NET INCREASE IN CASH & CASH EQUIVALENTS	=====	$119,500
CASH & CASH EQUIVALENTS, BEGINNING OF YEAR		50,000
CASH & CASH EQUIVALENTS, END OF YEAR	_____	$169,500

Key Concepts

- Basic cash management tools in any medical facility include the petty cash fund, the cash drawer, and the proper operation of the operating checking account for both cash receipts and cash disbursements.

- The bank reconciliation will ensure that the accounting records of the medical facility for the operating checking account and the bank records for that account stay in agreement. Modern computer software assists in automating the process of bank reconciliation.

- The statement of cash flows supplements the information provided in the balance sheet and income statement, providing valuable information on where the medical facility generates cash and what that cash is used for.

Investing, Borrowing, and the Time Value of Money

Chapter 10

Key Terms

The American Recovery and Reinvestment Act (ARRA) of 2009

Balloon maturity

Bonds

Credit risk

Federal Deposit Insurance Corporation (FDIC)

Fixed rate

Foreign exchange risk

Government policy risk

Inflation

Interest

Interest rate risk

Issuer

Line of credit

London Interbank Offered Rate (LIBOR)

Par value

Rule of 72

Security

Single payment loan

Term loan

Time value of money

Variable rate

Chapter Objectives

After completing this chapter, readers should be able to:

- Apply principles of the time value of money to calculations in financial mathematics.

- Discuss banking relationships and how disruptions in the financial markets will affect the relationships.

- Describe the safe and prudent investment of cash not needed immediately to support operations.

- Explain the types of bank loans available to medical facilities and the uses of each.

- Identify the use of bonds for major financings.

Chapter Glossary

The American Recovery and Reinvestment Act (ARRA) of 2009 was approved as a stimulus for capital investment. The act included funding for computerized medical records in a standardized format.

Balloon maturity is an exceptionally large single payment due at a fixed date in the future.

Bonds are securities (see term later in this list) where the issuer borrows money from an investor and promises to repay the investor a fixed principal and interest at a stated rate on a specific date.

Credit risk is the danger that the value of a security held will fall with declines in the financial strength of the company issuing the security.

Federal Deposit Insurance Corporation (FDIC) is the federal agency insuring bank deposits for individual investors.

Fixed rate on a loan or security denotes that the interest rate will remain constant or change only on a predetermined schedule.

Foreign exchange risk is the danger in investing in foreign securities that the value of a security will be worth less in U.S. dollars if the currency exchange rate changes.

Government policy risk is the danger that the value of a security will fall based on changes in policy by the government in the country where the security is issued.

Inflation is the increase over time of the general level of costs of goods and services in the economy.

Interest is the cost incurred to borrow money or the payment received to loan or invest money.

Interest rate risk is the danger that the value of a security will fall if market interest rates increase.

Issuer in a bond offering is the legal entity borrowing the funds and agreeing to repayment terms.

Line of credit is an agreement allowing for draw up to a maximum amount in a certain period of time.

London Interbank Offered Rate (LIBOR) is an accepted standard as a benchmark for variable rate loans and investments.

Par value is the original stated price, or face amount, of the investment or bond.

The **Rule of 72** is an easy method to determine the number of years required for an investment to double in value at fixed annual rates of interest.

A **security** is a financial instrument that represents either financial ownership (corporate stocks) or a debt agreement (bonds or banking agreements with an interest rate and a fixed maturity date).

Single payment loan is a bank loan for a specific period of time with one payment at maturity.

Term loan is a bank loan over an extended period of time with required periodic payments.

The **time value of money** is the concept of interest that a dollar available today is worth more than a dollar received in the future.

Variable rate on a loan or security means that the interest rate will adjust periodically based on an index.

Introduction

America's financial markets impact everyone's daily lives. A technician at the local hospital drives to work in the morning, stopping to fill her car with gas and using a debit card linked to her checking account. The car was purchased with a loan from the hospital's credit union. She has direct deposit of her paycheck. The account balance in her checking account as well as her investment in a bank certificate of deposit (CD) is protected with **Federal Deposit Insurance Corporation (FDIC)** insurance. She makes monthly payments on a student loan that financed her professional training and has her monthly mortgage payment automatically paid from her checking account. She has a 401(k) plan through the hospital invested in a stock mutual fund.

Just as individuals rely on the smooth operations of the financial markets, so do all businesses. The business checking account is just the most obvious connection to the financial markets. Chapter 11, Revenue Cycle Management, discusses effective ways to expedite the cash flow of the medical facility. The end result of the cash flow process is either positive cash flow in excess of what is needed to support the daily operations of the facility or times when cash flow is not sufficient to support operations or for capital investment.

When the facility generates cash balances that are not needed immediately, those funds need to be invested in a way that will generate investment income safely and without severely limiting the facility's access to those invested funds. In cases where the facility encounters times when cash flow is not sufficient to cover operating costs, a loan relationship is needed to provide funds to meet this short-term cash deficit. Borrowing may also be required when the medical facility is forecasting the need for major capital investments, such as the purchase of expensive medical equipment or expansion or renovation of buildings. This chapter will cover the time value of money and the impacts of both positive and negative cash flow.

Large hospitals and multifacility holding companies will have significant financial reserves and will use either in-house investment professionals or outside financial advisors to manage investment portfolios. The responsibility for cash management in smaller medical facilities will fall to the manager or finance staff. While most medical professionals work in areas other than finance, a basic understanding of investment markets is beneficial to understanding the financial management of medical facilities.

The Time Value of Money

The **time value of money** is the concept of **interest**: a dollar available today is worth more than a dollar received in the future. A local bank is offering 1-year certificates of deposit at an annual interest rate of 2 percent. For each dollar invested, the lender will receive $1.02 a year later. The 2 cents represents interest on the investment. Given current interest rates, $1 today has the same value as $1.02 will have in 1 year. Conversely, that same bank is offering to make 1-year loans to qualified borrowers at an annual interest rate of 4 percent. For each dollar borrowed, $1.04 needs to be repaid in a year. The 4 cents represents interest paid on the loan.

The Rule of 72

The **rule of 72** is the simplest of financial mathematics. It is an easy way to estimate the approximate number of years required for an investment to double in value at specified annual interest rates, compounded annually. The number 72 is divided by the annual interest rate to determine the number of years required for the investment to double in value. If the annual interest rate is 6 percent, 72 is divided by 6 to yield 12 as the number of years for the investment to double.

Key Chapter Equation: Rule of 72

The rule of 72 equation is:
72/Annual Interest Rate = Years for Investment to Double

Future Values and Present Values

Cash is a commodity, and like other commodities it can be bought and sold. The price for this commodity of cash is expressed in terms of the interest rate that can be earned on funds invested or paid for cash when funds are borrowed. If a business has cash that can be invested for a certain period of time at interest rates available today, what will be the value of the investment at maturity? If a business has a fixed payment that needs to be made at a certain point in the future, how much cash needs to be set aside today to meet that payment?

Future values and present values are the financial mathematics used in these calculations and for a variety of other basic business financial questions. Formulas and tables of values for basic business computations are available to answer these questions. As a teaching tool, written formulas and published future and present value tables are used. In the real world, business calculators replaced manual computations long ago. Business calculators have in turn been replaced by Internet sites easily accessed through a web browser searching for "future value computation" or "present value computation."

The Future Value of a Single Sum

A common business question is to calculate the future value of a single sum of cash invested today. The future value of a single sum of cash equation is used.

Key Chapter Equation: Future Value of a Single Sum of Cash

The future value of a single sum of cash equation is:

f = p × f(i,n)

In this equation, **f** is the future value of the single sum invested today, **p** is the dollar amount invested at present, **i** is the rate of interest on the investment, and **n** is the number of periods, generally in years of investment.

Figure 10-1 is a segment of a future value table. The full table will have interest rates ranging from one-fourth of 1 percent to 12 percent across the top and have the number of periods along the left side ranging from 1 to 50. Full tables may be found on websites such as www.accountingformanagement.org or www.principlesofaccounting.com. Full tables will have values to four or five decimal places. Only three decimal places are used in this example.

PERIOD	1%	2%	4%	6%
5	1.051	1.104	1.217	1.338
6	1.062	1.126	1.265	1.419
7	1.072	1.149	1.316	1.504
8	1.083	1.172	1.369	1.594
9	1.940	1.195	1.423	1.689
10	1.105	1.219	1.480	1.791

© Cengage Learning 2013

Figure 10-1 A Partial Future Value Table

Example 10-1

The chief executive officer of St. Mary's Hospital receives a call from a local attorney notifying them that the hospital has been named in the will of a recently deceased client in the amount of $200,000. The hospital's board of trustees decides to use the bequest to fund the purchase of a new bloodmobile when the current vehicle reaches the end of its useful life in an estimated 6 years. The local bank is willing to offer the hospital a 6-year CD at an interest rate of 4 percent, compounded annually. How much will the hospital have available at the time of maturity of the investment? Using the future value of a single sum of cash equation:

$$f = p \times f(i,n)$$

$200,000 is the p for the present value and 1.265 is the value from the future value table for f(i,n) in Figure 10-1 for the intersection of 4 percent interest for 6 years. Thus:

$$\text{Future Value} = \$200,000 \times 1.265$$

At the end of 6 years at 4 percent annual interest, St. Mary's Hospital will have $253,000 for the purchase of the new bloodmobile, assuming no tax liability from the interest earned.

The Present Value of a Single Sum

A business needs to know how much money would need to be invested today to meet a financial obligation in the future. The present value of a single sum equation is used.

Key Chapter Equation: Present Value of a Single Sum

The present value of a single sum equation is:
$$p = f \times p(i,n)$$

In this equation, **p** is the dollar amount invested at present, **f** is the future value of the single sum, **i** is the rate of interest on the investment, and **n** is the number of periods, generally in years, of investment.

Figure 10-2 is a segment of a present value table.

PERIOD	1%	2%	4%	6%
5	0.951	0.906	0.822	0.747
6	0.942	0.888	0.790	0.705
7	0.933	0.871	0.760	0.665
8	0.923	0.853	0.731	0.627
9	0.914	0.837	0.703	0.592
10	0.905	0.820	0.676	0.558

© Cengage Learning 2013

Figure 10-2 A Partial Present Value Table

Example 10-2

Three years ago, Tall Pines Life Care Facility expanded their facility to add a secure area dedicated to patients with dementia. They negotiated a 10-year loan with affordable monthly payments and a lump-sum payment of $400,000 due at the end of the loan. How much would Tall Pines have to invest in cash today to meet the $400,000 payment in 7 years, assuming cash could be invested at 4 percent? Using the present value of a single sum equation:

$$p = f \times p(i,n)$$

$400,000 is the f for the future value and 0.760 is the value from the present value table for p(i,n) in Figure 10-2 for the intersection of 4 percent interest for 7 years. Thus:

$$\text{Present Value} = \$400,000 \times 0.760$$

Tall Pines would have to invest $304,000 today at 4 percent interest, compounded annually, to have $400,000 available in 7 years.

Banking Relationships

"There is a strong link between financial literacy and our other economic objectives. All markets function best when participants are educated. As Chairman Greenspan stated in recent Senate testimony on this subject, 'An informed borrower is simply less vulnerable to fraud and abuse'."

Remarks by Federal Reserve Governor Edward M. Gramlich at the Financial Literacy Teacher Training Workshop, University of Illinois at Chicago, May 2, 2002 www.federalreserve.gov/boarddocs/speeches/2002.

Banking relationships are as varied as medical facilities. The professional finance staff of a large hospital or hospital holding company will prepare a request for proposals (RFP) outlining the services that the medical facility expects the commercial bank to provide and will ask that the banks formally respond to the RFP with a banking proposal, affirming the bank's ability to meet the service requirements in the RFP and detailing both the bank's charges for services and the rate of interest that the bank will pay. In the bank's response, charges for service will generally be expressed in a fixed charge for each item processed, such as checks cleared and wire transfers. The interest to be paid on depository funds with the bank will generally be expressed as a percentage of a benchmark, such as the federal funds rate. The federal funds rate is the rate at which banks may borrow or lend funds between banks within the Federal Reserve System. If the current federal funds rate is 2 percent annualized and the bank is offering the customer an interest rate on deposits of the federal funds rate less one-half of 1 percent, the customer will earn 1.5 percent on balances in the account. Interest paid on the account will change as the federal funds rate changes based on economic conditions.

The medical facility's finance staff will review the banking proposals received, calculate the annual cost of banking services, and interview those banks most responsive to the RFP. The final decision on the award of a banking services contract will commonly come down to customer service considerations and technological improvements offered by one of the competing banks. As in all other industries, the computer has revolutionized banking services, and banks are anxious to show their latest advances. As an example, one of the improvements implemented over the past decade has been a computer program to prevent the fraudulent forging or altering of checks issued by the medical facility. With each week's accounts payable batch run, the facility will upload to the bank's computer system a file with the check numbers and amounts. Prior to clearing any of the facility's checks, the bank will match data from the uploaded file to the checks presented for payment. When competing banks have similar fee schedules, enhancements such as this can determine where the facility chooses to place their business. The bank's reputation for customer service can best be measured by contacting current customers. A professional RFP will include the requirement to list several customers similar to the organization issuing the RFP, including the name and phone number of the bank's primary contact at the reference. As part of the review process of the proposals received, references will be called with particular attention paid to issues such as the efficiency and friendliness in conducting routine banking and in the ability of the bank's relationship manager to successfully handle any issues that may arise during the contract.

Case Study 10-1

Summit Regional Medical Center operates as a private not-for-profit hospital, providing services to a community of 20,000 and the surrounding rural areas. Summit has maintained a banking relationship with the local community bank for decades, and a number of individuals on the hospital's board of directors are local businesspeople who also maintain relationships with the local bank. Physicians and administrative staff of the hospital have developed a report showing that major pieces of medical equipment have become outdated by recent improvements in technology and need to be replaced. A financial review shows that new patient revenues from the use of the equipment will repay the capital investment over 5 years. The board of directors approves the purchases, and the hospital's finance director schedules a meeting with the bank's vice-president. The banker reports that due to an increase in nonperforming loans in the current recession and slow recovery, the bank cannot make the $1 million loan to the hospital. Another bank in the community is a branch of a major national banking system. When approached, that bank states that they only make new loans to established customers but indicates that if all of the banking relationship were to be transferred from the community bank to the national bank, the loan would be approved.

What action should the hospital's finance director and chief executive officer make to the board?

For smaller medical facilities, the process tends to be much simpler. The physician plays golf with a banker at the local country club or the practice manager has a series of informal meetings with banks in the area. While simpler, the decision on a banking services provider has important considerations for the facility. Banks can fail. The local independent bank may be bought out by a major national bank and the personal relationship developed lost. In the recent severe economic recession, the ability of many banks to make new loans was limited by their exposure to bad real-estate loans. Whereas in previous years the facility could shop their loan request for the best rate, many banks restrict new loans to established customers in times of tight credit, if they have the ability to make new loans at all. A large number of banks did not survive the recession.

Figure 10-3 shows the total assets and bank failures from 2001 through 2022. The total number of bank failures was 561 during this time period.

Medical facilities, large and small, need to develop effective banking relationships. This can be done by either strengthening an existing relationship or building a new one. Most banks will assign a relationship manager to each business account. The relationship manager needs to be kept informed of the financial status of the medical facility. The facility, to the extent that the bank is competitive on fees, should consolidate deposits, investments, credit cards, and loans with a single commercial bank. In times of economic contraction, how strongly established a banking relationship is will determine future access to funds needed by the medical facility. On its part, it is the responsibility of the medical facility to stay current with information on the financial status of the bank. Many banking records are on the public record and can easily be accessed through the Internet.

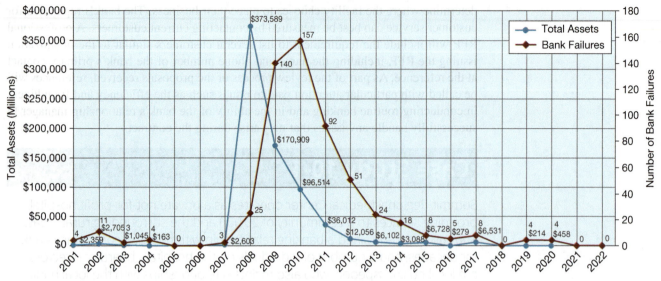

Figure 10-3 Number of Bank Failures

Knowledge Check 10.1

1. In Case Study 10-1, Summit Regional Health Center is faced with a dilemma. They can either maintain ties to the local bank and postpone the major capital acquisition or move all of their banking business to a new bank, a branch of a major national banking system. The board of directors of the bank has been informed of the issues and has requested that you, as the chief financial officer of the hospital, prepare a report for the board's consideration, outlining the issues involved and the options available, and forward a recommendation. What items would you consider to be relevant, and what recommendation would you make to the board?

_____

_____

_____

2. The finance department of a large hospital negotiates banking services with a 3-year contract. Nearing the end of the contract period, which of the following will be used to determine the award of a new 3-year banking services contract?
   A. Informal written bids
   B. Request for proposal
   C. Telephone bids

3. Which of the following will negatively impact the relationship between a medical facility and a bank?
   A. Deterioration in the financial condition of the medical facility
   B. The bank reporting major losses from nonperforming loans
   C. Disruptions in national and international financial markets
   D. All of the above

Available Funds

Money is available for investment when the cash flow of a medical facility generates funds that are not needed immediately to meet financial obligations. These funds may be invested in a wide variety of corporate and government securities. A **security** is a financial instrument that represents either financial ownership (corporate stocks) or a debt agreement (bonds or banking agreements with an interest rate and a fixed maturity date). Examples would include the stock of a publicly held corporation traded on a major stock exchange, U.S. Treasury bills, notes, and bonds, and bank deposits with a fixed interest rate and maturity date.

Example 10-3

The Oncology Centers operate a number of outpatient cancer treatment centers throughout the metropolitan area. Two years ago, they entered into a loan agreement in the amount of $560,000 to upgrade radiation equipment. The loan is for a period of 7 years at the fixed interest rate of 7 percent. Annual payments are $80,000 plus interest on the outstanding balance. There is no prepayment penalty on the loan. After 2 years of payments, the loan balance is $400,000. Over those 2 years, positive cash flow has resulted in a balance in the bank operating account of $200,000 more than required operating reserves. Rachel Smithson, finance manager for the Oncology Centers, has forecasted that positive cash flow over the next 18 months will allow for the loan to be fully paid. Ms. Smithson meets with her relationship manager at the bank to discuss investment options. The banker gives her the following options:

1. A 18-month bank CD yielding 1.5 percent annually

2. A 10-year U.S. Treasury note yielding 2.75 percent interest

3. A Federal Home Loan Bank (FHLB) 5-year step-up note. The interest rate on the note is 1 percent for the first year, 1.25 percent for the second year, and 3.5 percent for the remaining 3 years. The agency can call the note at any time at par.

Where should Ms. Smithson invest the $200,000? The prudent investment of available funds is more complicated than simply investing in the security with the highest available interest rate and hoping that economic conditions will not impact the value of the security.

Funds that are not needed immediately to support the operations of the business are invested to generate investment income until such time as the funds are needed. Investors are faced with a myriad of investment choices, each with its own benefits and drawbacks. Funds that will be needed at a known point in the future for a specific purpose, such as the purchase of capital equipment or for facility expansion, will be invested differently than funds that provide emergency reserves for the business. Generally, the longer the term of an investment, the higher the rate of interest. Funds needed at a specific point in the future should be invested so that the investments mature near the time the funds are needed to ensure that the investor will receive a set amount on the maturity of the investment.

The prudent investment of business funds dictates that funds are invested short-term in low-risk investment instruments. The downside of this prudence is that the investor has to accept investment returns that are lower than placing funds in longer-term, higher-risk investments. Smaller medical facilities will tend to keep their investments simple, while larger hospitals and some medical corporations will have the staff expertise to run sophisticated investment programs. For all medical facilities, it is important to remember that they are in the healthcare business, not the financial speculation business. Box 10-1 highlights three simple rules to remember in investing funds.

// Comprehension Check 10.1

1. Farrah Singh works at Ginhi Medical Facility within the finance department. Her supervisor asked her to outline the services that the medical facility expects when looking for a commercial bank and to search for various banks that can meet the organization's service requirements. What will Farrah have to prepare?

2. Farrah Singh will be reviewing the federal fund rate of each bank as well. Why is the federal fund rate important when determining the medical facility's banking needs?

BOX 10-1 Rules of Investing Funds

1. **Safety.** The safety of the principal invested is always the first consideration.

2. **Liquidity.** Funds are invested in securities that are readily marketable or may be surrendered without excessive fees if funds are needed sooner than expected.

3. **Yield.** The interest to be earned on the investment is an important consideration; however, it is always third in priority after safety and liquidity.

Short-Term, Low-Risk Investments

Finance managers have a variety of investment options available that meet the requirements of safety and liquidity:

- Bank certificates of deposits (CDs)
- U.S. Treasury bills, Treasury notes, and Treasury bonds
- Federal Agency Securities

Bank Certificates of Deposit (CDs)

Bank CDs are issued in a wide variety of denominations and maturities based on the need of the investor. CDs from chartered banks are insured up to $100,000 per depositor by the Federal Deposit Insurance Corporation (FDIC). The $100,000 is a total limit for all accounts of a single depositor and was increased to $250,000 during the recession of 2007–2009. The increased limit was designed to maintain investor confidence in bank deposits at a time when banks were faced with losses from real-estate loans. Interest on the CD may be paid periodically or at maturity.

U.S. Treasury Bills, Treasury Notes, and Treasury Bonds

The federal government is a major issuer of debt to finance the accumulated deficit of the country. Debt is issued with maturities from 91 days in a short-term treasury bill to 30 years in a treasury bond. Treasury bills are sold at a discount and mature at **par value**, while notes and bonds pay interest semiannually. The par value of any security is the original stated value of the instrument. The market value of a security is the price that the security trades at in the securities markets. There is an active market in federal securities, providing investors with a wide variety of available maturity dates for investments. This provides investors with the opportunity to select an investment with a maturity date that coincides with the need for access to funds. Guaranteed by the full faith and credit of the federal government as to both principal and interest, treasury obligations are accepted as a global safe haven for cash. Banks and brokerage houses provide access to these markets, and investors may deal directly with the federal government on purchases of new issue securities.

Federal Agency Securities

A wide variety of federal agencies issue an even wider variety of securities to finance lending operations. Securities range from short-term 30-day securities to 30-year mortgage pools. These agencies include the Governmental National Mortgage Association (GNMA, called "Ginnie Mae"), the Federal Home Loan Mortgage Corporation (FHLMC, called "Freddie Mac"), and the Federal National Mortgage Association (FNMA called "Fannie Mae"). With the exception of GNMA securities, which are fully guaranteed by the federal government as to both principal and interest, agency securities are not full-faith-and-credit obligations of the federal government. Financial markets treat non-insured agency securities as having an "implied guarantee" against default and will carry interest rates higher than similar maturity guaranteed treasuries but lower than high-grade corporate securities. As with treasuries, agency securities may be purchased from banks or brokerage houses.

Three Major Principles of Investing Funds

The successful investing of available funds is based on three principles:

- The time value of money is based on the concept of interest.
- Prudent investing requires understanding the markets and securities.
- Investors are rewarded for the risks they take.

The Time Value of Money

All financial markets exist on the premise that investors expect to receive more money back in the future than the amount that was originally invested. An investor purchases a bank CD for $10,000. When the certificate matures in 1 year, the bank pays $10,150. The $150 gain reflects the time value of money.

Prudent Investing Requires Understanding Markets and Securities

The golden rule for investors is, "If you don't understand it, don't buy it." Back in more expansive economic times, prior to the bursting of the high-tech bubble in 2000 and the real-estate bubble in 2007, exotic investments were packaged and sold to investors. Many of these investments were purchased by unsophisticated investors who were unaware of the risks involved and suffered large portfolio losses. The individual charged with the responsibility of investing the organization's funds must ensure that every potential investment is fully understood and the risks known.

Investors Are Rewarded for Risks Taken

The 1-year bank CD discussed earlier paid interest at the rate of 1.5 percent annually. Since the bank CD was insured by the FDIC, the risk to the investor from loss of principal is not an issue. A 10-year treasury note, also considered to be a risk-free investment backed by the full faith and credit of the federal government, will pay interest at the annual rate of 3 percent, with interest payments made semiannually. Many corporate bonds will carry interest rates in excess of 5 percent. Several factors are involved in investment risk:

Interest rate risk. The basic tool used by the federal government to attempt to either stimulate or suppress economic activity is the control of the money supply. To assist the economy to recover from a recession, the government will make access to funds easier, bringing down interest rates and promoting capital investment and economic expansion. When the economy is strong, tightening the money supply will increase interest rates and serve to hold down inflationary pressures. Changes in market interest rates impact investors. A new-issue 10-year treasury note is purchased with a stated interest rate of 3 percent. Two years later, when the economy is beginning a strong recovery, the federal government has become more concerned with **inflation** than recession. A new-issue 10-year treasury note issued at that time carries an annual interest rate of 4 percent. The old 3 percent treasury note, with 8 years to maturity, cannot be competitive with a 3 percent interest yield and the financial markets will price the 3 percent treasury note at a discount. The amount of the discount must be sufficient to compensate a new purchaser of the old bond for accepting a below-market interest rate for the remaining life of the old bond. The new purchaser of the discounted old bond will receive interest payments of 3 percent of the face value of the bond for the life of the bond and will then receive the face value at maturity.

BOX 10-2 Federal Interest Rates

Interest rates will move in both directions, up and down. Federal actions to reduce interest rates to stimulate the economy provided gains for investors holding bonds issued before the recession. In February 2001, the U.S. Treasury issued a series of 30-year bonds at an interest rate of 5.375 percent. Due to declining interest rates, the June 2011 value of this bond was 120, a 20 percent gain for investors who had purchased the investment in 2001 at par.

Credit risk. Purchasers of corporate bonds rely on the creditworthiness of the company issuing the bonds rather than the full faith and credit of the federal government available for treasury issues or FDIC insurance available (subject to limits) for bank certificates of deposit. The interest rates on new corporate bond issues with similar maturities will vary based on the analysis of the financial markets as to their ability to pay off the debt at the maturity in the future. A strong industrial company issues 20-year bonds for plant expansion at par in 2004 at an annual interest rate of 6 percent. During the severe recession of 2007 to 2009, the company experiences financial difficulties and is forced to file for bankruptcy reorganization. In 2010, any investor looking to purchase these 6 percent bonds with 14 years left to maturity will demand a large premium in the form of a discounted purchase price to compensate for the risk of default on the bonds. The original purchaser of these bonds at par would experience a major loss on the bonds if sold in 2010. Conversely, if the company returns to profitability and redeems the bonds at par at maturity, a buyer of deeply discounted bonds would experience a large gain on the investment.

Comprehension Check 10.2

Answer the following questions based on investment of funds.

1. Define what a market value is.

2. What are three major principles of investing funds?

3. How does the federal government control the money supply?

BOX 10-3 Casualty of a Bond Market

For decades, General Motors Corporation was a fixture of American industry, building automobiles and operating related businesses. GM was an active participant in the bond market, using bonds to raise funds for capital investment. GM was one of the largest casualties of the recent recession. The company declared bankruptcy in June 2009. At the time of the declaration of bankruptcy, GM's bonds were trading on the securities markets at a value between 30 and 35 percent of the original par value of the bonds. Investors who had purchased GM bonds at par lost more than two-thirds of the value of their investments.

Foreign exchange risk and **government policy risk**. Sophisticated investors purchasing foreign securities deal with risk factors beyond interest rate risk and credit risk. The changing relationship between the U.S. dollar and the foreign currency of the security purchased will impact the dollar value of the security. Unstable foreign governments may reduce the value of securities issued in that country.

Knowledge Check 10.2

1. An investor purchases a 10-year U.S. Treasury note and then wishes to sell the investment after 2 years. During those 2 years, interest rates for all investments have dropped from the market rates available when the investment was purchased. At the time of sale, what would the investment be worth?
A. More than the purchase price of the investment
B. Less than the purchase price of the investment
C. The same as the purchase price of the investment
D. Insufficient information is provided to determine the answer

2. Which of the following investments are guaranteed by the federal government?
A. Government National Mortgage Association (GNMA) securities
B. Federal Home Loan Bank (FHLB) notes
C. U.S. Treasury notes
D. An individual's bank account balances totaling $82,000
E. All of the above
F. All of the above except A
G. All of the above except B

Insufficient Cash Flow to Meet Obligations

The need to borrow money is a condition faced by many medical facilities. Proceeds of borrowing are used to expand facilities, to upgrade major pieces of equipment, and sometimes to meet operating needs. Commercial banks are the source of borrowing for the great majority of medical facilities. Large hospital corporations have access to other forms of financing, such as issuing additional stock in the corporation or selling taxable corporate bonds. Facilities operated by state and local governments, as well as medical facilities operated in the public interest, are able to issue tax-exempt bonds.

Commercial Banks

Commercial banks serve the borrowing needs for most medical facilities. There are a number of types of commercial bank loans available:

- Single payment loan
- Line of credit
- Terms loan

Single Payment Loan

A **single payment loan** at a stated interest rate, calling for a single repayment at a certain date, is the most basic source of needed funds. A local hospital has purchased a piece of capital equipment and is comfortable that positive cash flow over the next several months will provide the cash to pay for the purchase. The hospital negotiates a single payment bank loan with a fixed rate of interest, payable in 90 days.

Line of Credit

In a **line of credit** arrangement, the medical facility and the bank negotiate an agreement whereby the medical facility is allowed to draw funds from the bank up to a maximum amount over a stated period of time. Once the agreement has been approved, each individual draw on the line of credit is handled with a minimum of paperwork. Interest rates on a line of credit may be either at a fixed rate or on a variable rate based on an accepted index, such as the **prime rate**. The prime rate is the interest rate charged by a bank on loans to its best customers. Interest rates charged to nonprime borrowers will be higher than the prime rate. During the life of the agreement, the medical facility will draw funds as needed for items such as capital equipment or to meet times of negative cash flow. Positive cash flow at a later date allows the medical facility to pay down all or part of the outstanding balance on the line of credit, allowing for future draws. At the expiration date of the agreement, a new line of credit may be negotiated or any remaining balance transferred to a new fixed loan.

//// Comprehension Check 10.3

1. Savannah Medical Facility for hospital renovations needs to arrange with a local bank to draw funds for up to 100,000 for 10 years. This is an example of what type of credit arrangement with the bank?

2. Pearson Dental needs to purchase new laser dental equipment. The dental practice is seeking 85,000 for 5 years at a fixed rate of interest. This is an example of what type of credit arrangement with the bank?

Case Study 10-2

Drs. Draper and Keys run a partnership family medical practice in Brownsville, Texas. While the practice is profitable, both physicians are making payments on heavy debt loads for student loans that financed their medical training. A significant percentage of their patient base is made up of "Winter Texans," retirees from America's heartland who choose to winter in a warmer climate. The positive cash flow in the winter months is more than sufficient to offset negative cash flow during the slower summer months. The permanent staff of the practice is needed to support operations during the winter months, and the partners do not want to lose trained and effective staff members from layoffs during the summer months. They have tried using part-time employees during the winter months; however, the local economy does not have a pool of trained medical staff available for part-time work. The partners have met with their local banker to discuss this seasonal problem.

What would be an effective solution for the banker to recommend?

Term Loans

Term loans are bank loans for an extended period of time, normally at least 2 years, and generally with a fixed repayment schedule and a fixed rate of interest. This type of loan is very similar to an individual purchasing an automobile and financing the purchase over a number of years with a fixed monthly payment based on the negotiated interest rate. Medical facilities will generally use this type of loan for a major asset purchase and may be required by the bank to pledge the asset as security for repayment of the loan.

Case Study 10-3

Dr. Cynthia Bower operates a successful family medical practice. She has a loyal patient base, but sometimes is not able to schedule patients when they wish to be seen. She rents office space in a medical professional building. The adjacent office suite becomes vacant, and Dr. Bower thinks that this may be a good time to expand the practice by bringing in a partner and doubling the size of the rented office space. She discusses the idea with Tim McGuire, her office manager, and the two of them develop a plan to finance the expansion, with revenues from the expanded business providing funds to meet increased operating expenses and debt service. The initial capital investment to prepare the new office space for a second physician is estimated at $500,000.

They meet with the practice's relationship manager at First National Bank to discuss a bank loan to cover the costs of expansion. The relationship manager reviews the plan and agrees that the revenues generated by the second physician will comfortably cover the increased operating expenses and debt service on a loan. The bank's loan committee agrees to approve the loan but does not wish the loan to extend for more than 5 years, given the current economic conditions. Dr. Bower and the bank agree to a 5-year bank note with affordable payments and a **balloon maturity** payment due at the end of 5 years.

A balloon maturity payment incorporated into a loan repayment schedule is a single, unusually large payment to settle the balance of the loan outstanding. Positive cash flow over the next 5 years may provide sufficient cash to pay the balloon maturity payment; if not, the amount of the balloon maturity payment

continued

will need to be refinanced when the payment is due. The approved loan calls for semiannual principal and interest payments, with the interest rate at 7 percent on the balance outstanding. The loan closes on October 31, 2010, with the following repayment schedule:

DATE	PRINCIPAL	INTEREST	PAYMENT
4/30/2011	$20,000	$17,500	$37,500
10/31/2011	20,000	16,800	36,800
4/30/2012	25,000	16,100	41,100
10/31/2012	25,000	15,225	40,225
4/30/2013	30,000	14,350	44,350
10/31/2013	30,000	13,300	43,300
4/30/2014	35,000	12,250	47,250
10/31/2014	35,000	11,025	46,025
4/30/2015	40,000	9,450	49,450
10/31/2015	240,000	8,050	248,050
TOTALS	$500,000	$134,050	$634,050

© Cengage Learning 2013

Bank Note Schedule

Do you agree that expanding the business is a financially prudent action for Dr. Bower? Explain how you arrived at your conclusion.

Corporate and Tax-Free Municipal Bonds

Banks provide access to needed funds for smaller medical facilities. For larger healthcare providers, such as major urban hospitals, hospital holding companies, and hospitals that are owned by local governments through a governmental hospital authority, the bond market serves as an efficient source of funds. **Bonds** represent long-term promises to pay and are backed by the creditworthiness of the issuing entity.

Bonds issued or guaranteed by federal agencies such as the GNMA are backed by the "full faith and credit of the U.S. government," just like Treasuries. This is an unconditional commitment to pay interest payments and to return the principal investment in full to you when a debt security reaches maturity.

Bonds issued by GSEs such as FNMA, FHLMC, and The Federal Agricultural Mortgage Corporation ("Farmer Mac") are not backed by the same guarantee as federal government agencies. Bonds issued by GSEs carry credit risk.

The **issuer** of the bonds is the legal entity borrowing the funds and contractually obligated to meet the debt service requirements on the bonds. Bonds are generally issued in $5,000 denominations, with a set number of the bonds maturing each year during the life of the bond issue. Bonds maturing in the early years of the issue will carry a lower interest rate than the bonds maturing later in the issue.

A for-profit hospital holding company may issue taxable bonds to finance new hospital acquisitions. With taxable bonds, the bondholder is required to report the interest received on the bonds to the IRS as taxable income. More commonly, not-for-profit hospitals will issue bonds to build or expand their facilities. Under the federal income tax code, state and local government agencies are able to issue bonds with interest payments that are exempt from federal income taxes and may also be exempt from state taxes. The tax exemption allows these governments to issue bonds at a lower interest rate than if the interest were taxable income to the holder of the bonds. Further legislation has extended the tax-exempt status of the bonds to qualified medical facilities acting in the public interest. These are referred to as **conduit bonds** and provide medical facilities with the same tax-exempt status on interest paid on the bonds as the bonds issued directly by the local governments.

Example 10-4

St. John's Hospital serves the medical needs of a community of 40,000 people in Kentucky. It is chartered as a tax-exempt nonprofit hospital as St. John's Hospital Authority. The hospital enjoys a favorable reputation in the community and is in strong financial condition. The board of directors, at the recommendation of hospital management, has agreed to a major renovation of the aging facility. The hospital has worked with the outside financial advisors and architects, determining the costs of the renovation and structuring a tax-exempt bond issue to provide the needed financing. The hospital's cash flow is sufficient to handle the debt service, and the bonds will be paid off over a period of 10 years. The proposed debt service schedule, with interest rates based on current market conditions, is shown in Figure 10-4.

$6,250,000
St. John's Hospital Authority
Facility Improvement Revenue Bonds
Series 2010

Maturity (October 1)	Principal Amount	Interest Rate
2011	$520,000	1.90%
2012	540,000	2.10%
2013	560,000	2.25%
2014	575,000	2.50%
2015	615,000	2.70%
2016	630,000	2.90%
2017	660,000	3.10%
2018	685,000	3.30%
2019	710,000	3.60%
2020	755,000	3.90%

© Cengage Learning 2013

Figure 10-4 Bond Maturities Schedule

Participants in the Bond Process

Using the example of a tax-exempt municipal bond issue, the major players involved in structuring the bond issue and raising funds for the organization include:

- The **issuer** of the bonds is the healthcare organization looking to raise funds in the bond market.

- The issuer will generally retain the services of a **financial advisor**. The financial advisor will work with the issuer on structuring the bond and preparing the financial data to be provided to rating agencies and bond insurers.

- The bond **underwriter** is a securities dealer responsible for bringing the bonds to market. The underwriter assumes a financial risk by purchasing the bonds at less than the expected market value of the bonds (the underwriter's discount). As an example, the healthcare financing authority of a state government wishes to raise $100 million for the expansion of several hospitals in the state. A bond underwriter is hired through an RFP process. The underwriter assists in structuring the maturities of the bond issue to obtain the lowest market interest rates for the issuer. The underwriter agrees to purchase all $100 million of the bonds at a price of $4,975 per each $5,000 bond. The $25 difference per bond is the underwriter's discount. On the $100 million bond issue, the underwriter's discount is $500,000 before costs and the risks of holding the bonds until sold to investors or brokers. Risk is reduced by securing investor commitments to purchase bonds in advance of the sale date of the bonds and spreading the total amount of the bond between several underwriters. **Bond counsel** and **underwriter's counsel** are law firms that specialize in the legalities involved in bond issues.

- Bond **rating agencies** are paid a fee to assign a credit rating to the bond issue. The rating assigned informs potential purchasers of the financial strength of the issuer of the bonds and the likelihood that the issuer will make all of the scheduled debt payments over the life of the bond. Each individual bond issue will carry a credit rating at the time of the sale of the bonds, and the credit rating of the issuer will be updated through the life of the debt. Bonds are purchased by individual investors and by institutions, such as bond mutual funds. Bonds are divided into "investment grade" bonds and "junk" bonds. In the scales in Figure 10-4, "investment grade," required by many institutional purchasers, is BBB and above. A "junk bond" is a security with an investment rating lower than BBB. Bond ratings may change over time. A security that is originally issued by an organization with an investment grade rating may fall into junk bond territory when the organization experiences financial difficulties. The schedule given in Figure 10-5 shows the rating scales for the three major bond rating agencies.

BOND RATINGS:

STANDARD & POOR'S	MOODY'S	FITCH	
AAA	Aaa	AAA	Highest Credit Quality
AA	Aa	AA	Very High Credit Quality
A	A	A	High Credit Quality
BBB	Baa	BBB	Good Credit Quality
BB	Ba	BB	Speculative
B	B	B	Highly Speculative
CCC	Caa	CCC	Substantial Credit Risk
CC	Ca	CC	Very High Credit Risk
C	C	C	Exceptionally High Credit Risk
D	DDD	D	Default

© Cengage Learning 2013

Figure 10-5 Bond Ratings

- The higher the credit rating assigned to a bond issue, the lower the market interest rate. Since the 1970s, **bond insurance** has been available to provide a means for issuers to upgrade their bond ratings. Bond insurance companies, for a onetime premium payment, agree to step in to meet debt service payment obligations when the issuer does not have the financial ability to make the payments. Prior to collapse of the mortgage industry in 2007–2009, a majority of tax-free bond issues were marketed with bond insurance and the largest bond insurance companies carried a AAA credit rating. With the purchase of bond insurance, the AAA credit rating of the insurance company replaces the lower credit rating of the individual issuer as the credit quality of the bond issue, saving the issuer interest costs over the life of the bond. Bond insurance is purchased when the net present value of the lifetime savings on interest expense exceeds the premium for the purchase of the insurance. That analysis is traditionally performed by the financial advisor. Since 2007, the bond insurance companies insuring the majority of insured tax-free bond issues have been downgraded to less than AAA credit quality due to their exposure to losses in the mortgage industry. Issuers now need to consider the few AAA-rated bond insurance providers that remain or use an alternative strategy, such as marketing their bonds on an uninsured basis, relying on the credit rating of the issuer.

February 2021–The hospital and health system credit ratings are as follows:

S&P Global Ratings affirmed the "BBB" issuer credit rating on Seattle-based Virginia Mason Medical Center. The credit rating agency also revised the credit rating outlook from stable to positive. The affirmation and outlook revision is a result of Virginia Mason's deal to form an 11-hospital health system with CHI Franciscan, based in Tacoma, Washington. S&P views the merger as a positive for the medical center.

Moody's affirmed the "A3" rating of Shands Teaching Hospital and Clinics in Florida, affecting $841 million of rated debt. The affirmation reflects the hospital's role as an academic medical center for the University of Florida College of Medicine, which will help its enterprise growth, Moody's said. The outlook is stable.

Fitch affirmed Jupiter (Fla.) Medical Center's "BBB+" issuer default rating and "BBB+" revenue bond rating on its $32.1 million series 2013A. Fitch cited the medical center's leading market position in Jupiter and the completion of a new patient tower as credit strengths lending to the affirmation. The outlook is stable.

Nonprofit hospitals that are not chartered as hospital authorities and thus are not able to issue tax-exempt bonds directly are authorized by federal law to access the tax-free bond market with the use of **Industrial Development Revenue Bonds** (**IDRBs**). IDRBs were originally authorized by federal legislation as a mechanism where local governments could use tax-free bonds as enticement for industrial expansion in a local economy. Hospitals were considered to be of such importance to the economy of local communities that they were included in the legislation. With an IDRB, the local government serves as a **conduit issuer** of the bonds and the bonds will carry the name of the local government. However, the hospital is responsible for meeting debt service obligations on the bonds and the bonds carry the credit rating of the hospital.

The American Recovery and Reinvestment Act (ARRA) of 2009 was approved as a stimulus for capital investment as the country attempted to recover from the severe recession. This act included the creation of **Build America Bonds** (**BABs**), authorizing eligible government as well as nonprofit hospitals to issue taxable revenue bonds, with the federal treasury reimbursing the issuer 35 percent of the interest costs on the bonds. The 35 percent interest rebate, combined with the ability to purchase bond insurance from the Federal Housing Administration, made BABs an attractive alternative to standard tax–exempt bonds.

Fixed-Rate and Variable-Rate Debt

Bank loans and bonds may both be structured with either a fixed rate or a variable rate. With a **fixed-rate** debt instrument, the interest rate is set at the time of the completion of the debt and will not change to maturity. With a commercial bank loan, the bank will offer a proposed interest rate for the loan, and the borrower may accept the rate or attempt to negotiate a more favorable interest rate either with that bank or with a competing bank. In fixed-rate bond issues, bonds maturing each year will normally have different interest rates, with the shortest maturity bonds carrying the lowest interest rate and the longest maturity bonds carrying the highest interest rate. In a public bond issue, the interest rate for each annual maturity will be set by the financial markets when the bonds are sold.

With a **variable-rate** debt instrument, the interest rate will adjust periodically based on the formula and the index established in the debt instrument. The most widely accepted index worldwide is the **London Interbank Offered Rate (LIBOR)**. In addition to LIBOR as a benchmark for variable-rate debt, many banks use their prime lending rate for an index.

Example 10-5

A for-profit urban hospital has developed plans for a major renovation and expansion of its facility. The multimillion dollar construction project will take 18 months and will be financed with a long-term bond issue when construction is completed. The contract with the company doing the construction work calls for monthly progress payments. The CFO of the hospital meets with their bank's relationship manager and negotiates a line of credit to provide funds to pay the contractor. The loan is approved for the estimated total construction cost, with interest to be charged based on the daily LIBOR rate plus a negotiated adjustment factor. Interest is charged on the total of funds actually drawn by the hospital, not the approved total maximum amount of the loan. At the end of construction, the hospital will establish permanent financing and use the proceeds of the permanent financing to retire the line of credit.

Corporate Stock

For-profit hospital corporations looking to expand, either through the acquisition of other hospital entities or by expanding services within the same locality, will commonly finance the expansion with the issuance of corporate stock. Corporate stock represents the ownership equity in the corporation, as opposed to loans and bonds, which are shown on the balance sheet as debt. The largest of America's hospital corporations have millions of shares of stock issued, with total valuation of the corporation in the billions. Shares of stock of the corporation are actively traded on the nation's major stock exchanges such as the New York Stock Exchange.

Knowledge Check 10.3

1. In Case Study 10-2, Drs. Draper and Keys experience annual periods of negative cash flow and require infusions of cash to meet operating expenses. Their local bank will likely recommend to them a:
   A. Single payment loan
   B. Line of credit
   C. Term loan
   D. None of the above

2. Small businesses, such as single physician's practices and medical partnerships, will tend to do their borrowing with commercial banks. What criteria will the bank use to approve a loan to a small medical facility?

   _____

   _____

   _____

continued

3. When a medical facility applies for a commercial bank loan, they are required to complete the bank's standardized application package. Why does the bank require more than the annual financial reports prepared by the facility's outside accountant?

_____

_____

_____

4. A large urban hospital is chartered as a nonprofit. The hospital is looking to expand to better serve the local population. The hospital enjoys a strong financial position and can easily qualify for a traditional taxable mortgage. Why would the hospital use Industrial Development Revenue Bonds (IDRBs) instead?

_____

_____

_____

5. What is the advantage of purchasing bond insurance?

_____

_____

_____

6. Describe the role played by the underwriter in a bond issue.

_____

_____

_____

Key Concepts

- All medical facilities, regardless of size, need to develop effective banking relationships. The relationship is a two-way street, with the medical facility updating the bank on the facility's financial position while at the same time monitoring the health of the bank.

- Funds available over the level of prudent operating reserves need to be placed in secure investments that are highly liquid. Obtaining the highest interest rates is an important consideration, but safety and liquidity are the top priorities in selecting investments.

- When additional funds are required by a medical facility, structuring the borrowing is a function of the size of the medical facility. Smaller medical facilities will use their banking relationship for loans, while larger medical facilities will use the size and interest rate advantages of the bond market.

Revenue Cycle Management

Key Terms

Insurance contracts

Medical facility average cost

Medical facility marginal cost

Precertification

Private-pay patients

Revenue cycle management

Chapter Objectives

After completing this chapter, readers should be able to:

- Explain revenue cycle management: the process of collecting all funds owed to the medical facility, as quickly and easily as possible.

- Explain the seven steps in the claim process within a healthcare facility.

- Discuss the importance of written financial policies to assist in revenue cycle management.

- Describe the importance of ongoing staff training and workload management as tools in the process of collecting funds owed to the medical facility.

- Identify appropriate ways to deal with insurance companies and government programs.

- Describe revenue improvements from improved patient scheduling.

Chapter Glossary

Insurance contracts are legal agreements between the medical facility and an insurance company, detailing the terms of the agreement and specifying reimbursement rates for medical services.

Medical facility average cost is the total operating costs of the practice divided by the number of patient visits.

Medical facility marginal cost is the added cost to provide medical services for one additional patient visit.

Precertification is the requirement that the insurance company agree to the medical procedure in advance of service.

Private-pay patients are those patients who are responsible for the full financial costs of their medical care.

Revenue cycle management deals with the collection of the full amount of funds owed for medical services as quickly and efficiently as possible.

Introduction

Revenue cycle management deals with the collection of the full amount of funds owed for medical services as quickly and efficiently as possible. This process deals with getting money from other people and into the bank account of the medical facility. These revenues come from two sources: payments from patients, either as private pay or as deductibles and copayments, and payments from third parties such as insurance companies and government programs. Revenue cycle management includes best business practices that address the swift collection of funds due from either source.

Any business can find itself in a position where cash balances are not sufficient to pay the bills to operate the business. Net income may be strong, but net worth and accounts receivables are not cash and cannot be used to pay the bills. Whether as director of finance for a hospital or the practice manager for a single-physician medical office, the head of finance needs to actively manage cash flow to ensure that payments for services are received on a timely basis.

Most of this chapter is dedicated to the revenue cycle management program of physician and group practices. The subject is no less important for hospitals; however, the wide variety of types of medical services provided and the number of internal cost centers make revenue cycle analysis and the costing of medical services much more complex. Hospitals will generally have the benefit of a trained financial staff to deal with these issues.

Revenue cycle management includes the process from preregistration until the time patients do not pay, which enables the account to go into collections.

Figure 11-1 shows the process a claim goes through.

The following steps are what a claim process will go through within a healthcare facility.

1. Preregistration Process. Patient information is taken, the amount of insurance coverage is explained, and no-show policies are explained.

2. Registration. Patient information is verified. The forms are signed, and insurance coverage is provided.

3. Charge Capture. The payment comes from the patient, insurance companies, or the government.

4. Claim Submissions. The claim information is submitted to the insurance carrier.

5. Remittance Processing. This process determines what will be paid for services. Fee schedules are reviewed.

6. Insurance Follow-up. This process follows up on what has and has not been paid.

7. Collections. If a patient has a balance, a statement is sent out for payment every 30 days.

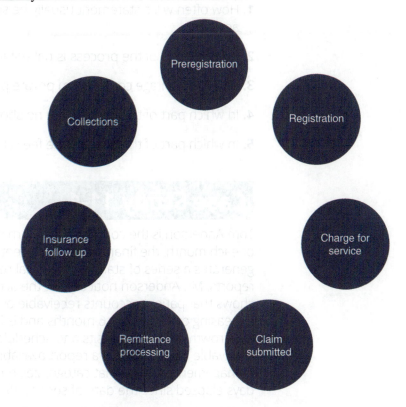

Figure 11-1 Revenue Cycle Management

Expediting Cash Flow on Patient Accounts

Increasing the speed of collection on customer accounts provides several benefits to the medical facility:

- More cash on hand provides funding to meet operating needs.

- Expediting cash flow may avoid the need for bank loans and related interest costs.

- The rate of collection on accounts receivables falls as the age of the receivable increases.

Financial Policies and Procedures

The medical industry is unique in how it receives payment for services. At the time of service, in many cases neither the medical facility nor the patient knows exactly who will be responsible for the payment of charges due. Only an estimated 3 percent to 3.5 percent of medical revenues come from **private-pay patients**, also referred to as self-pay patients, those who are responsible for the full costs of their medical care. The great majority of patients today are covered by healthcare insurance or government programs. As an example, a patient comes into a walk-in clinic with a laceration on his leg. The patient has a group medical plan that requires a $500 annual deductible and then a 20 percent copayment of the next $2,500. Facility personnel clean and stitch the laceration and bill the insurance company. The insurance company will pay the facility based on the contract rate for the specific service provided, less any deductible and copayment that remain the responsibility of the patient.

// Comprehension Check 11.1

1. How often will a statement usually be sent out if there is a balance on the account?

2. In which part of the process is patient information verified?

3. What percentage comes from private pay insurance?

4. In which part of the process are no shows explained?

5. In which part of the process are fee schedules discussed?

Case Study 11-1

Tom Anderson is the controller for Morningside Medical Clinic. At the end of each month, the financial management system used by Morningside generates a series of standard financial reports. In his review of the current reports, Mr. Anderson notices that the accounts receivable aging report shows that patient accounts receivable over 60 days old has been steadily increasing over the past 6 months and is increasing at a rate faster than the growth of inpatient visits and scheduled fees for services. An accounts receivable aging report is a report available in computerized financial management systems that categorizes receivables based on the number of days elapsed since the date of service. Receivables are grouped as:

- Receivables less than 30 days old
- Receivables between 31 and 60 days old
- Receivables more than 60 days old

This report serves as a measurement of the effectiveness of the medical facility's billing and collection procedures.

Morningside has detailed procedures in place to collect patient deductibles and copayments at time of service as well as procedures for billing account balances remaining after payments from insurance. Mr. Anderson calls a meeting with both employees responsible for receiving payments from customers at time of service and accounting personnel responsible for accounts receivable. The employees charged with the responsibility of receiving payments at time of service share an embarrassed look and admit that at times of high patient volume, they will sometimes tell patients that no payment is due simply to avoid delays at checkout. The accounts receivable clerks then share with Mr. Anderson how heavy their daily workload is and admit to neglecting to bill patients for balances due when other work needs to be completed. Mr. Anderson now understands the reasons behind the growth in accounts receivable balances.

What steps would be appropriate to resolve the problem?

Collection Policies and Procedures

Each different type of medical facility will have unique challenges and issues in the collection of funds due from patients. Every facility should have a set of written financial policies and procedures that deal with collection issues faced.

Establish a Payment Plan Before Service is Provided

Many medical facilities are able to schedule new patients far enough into the future to allow time for written communication with the patient regarding the patient's payment responsibilities. The facility sends the new patient a standard information package containing a form indicating the patient's signed acknowledgment of financial responsibility and the patient's agreement to pay at time of service. The facility will also verify with the patient's insurance company that the patient is a current member of the plan, that the medical procedure to be provided is covered, and take care of any **precertification** issues. Precertification is the requirement that the insurance company agree to the medical procedure in advance of service.

Collect at Time of Service

A common sight in medical offices is a discreet sign informing patients: **Payment Is Expected at Time of Service**. For many practices, this goes beyond the collection of the office visit copayment. The patient's full responsibility for deductibles and copayments may be estimated and that amount collected at time of service. Many facilities have now adopted a policy to request a credit card number from the patient. When the facility has received payment from insurance and the exact balance due from the patient is known, the patient's credit card is charged and the patient is provided with a courtesy call of the amount charged.

Verify Patient Information at Time of Service

As part of the check-in process for an appointment, the receptionist should verify the patient's address, telephone number(s), and insurance. The receptionist should ask, "Do you still live at … ?" rather than, "Have you moved?" Reciting the address will allow the patient to correct any errors in the facility's records. Annually or when there are any changes, the receptionist should photocopy the patient's insurance card to update the facility's records.

Billing Accounts Receivable

The patient should be billed for any balance due immediately upon receipt of payment from the insurance company, indicating the exact amount of the patient's financial responsibility. The patient will receive the bill from the facility at approximately the same time as the explanation of benefits (EOB) is received by the patient, confirming the amount due. If payment is not received from the patient within 30 days, the patient should be billed monthly until the balance has been paid. To smooth the office workload, batch and mail invoices on a weekly basis rather than billing all accounts at one time. The invoice from the facility should include a section indicating the status of the balance as to current, 30 days delinquent, 60 days delinquent, or 90+ days delinquent. For facilities billing with a color printer, highlighting the box for 90+ days delinquent in yellow is helpful. The billing should always include a contact phone number for patients with questions and a return envelope, which has proven to improve collections by a greater amount than the cost of the envelopes.

Have Flexible Payment Terms

A partial payment is better than no payment. Patients will experience financial difficulties, and the facility will need to be somewhat flexible in payment terms. Exceptions to the payment-at-time-of-service policy need to be clearly spelled out in the financial policies, including the staff position at the facility with the authority to approve exceptions. The facility should also have a form in place specifying the terms of accepting payments over a reasonable period of time. The patient and the facility agree to the repayment terms, and both sign the agreement. For the life of the agreement, payments need to be monitored, which requires staff time and should be used only as a last resort.

Patients on continuing care at a physician's office or an uninsured patient receiving hospital services can easily generate large outstanding account balances. The financial policies should establish a dollar limit that will automatically trigger a financial counseling session with the practice administrator or hospital financial counselor. The trigger amount can be as low as $2,500 or as high as $10,000, depending on the preferences of the facility.

Granting of Discounts

The granting of discounts for medical services can be an especially touchy subject. The conditions of appropriate use of discounts and the individuals authorized to grant discounts should be thoroughly disclosed in the financial policies.

Use of Collection Agencies and Considering Grounds for Dismissal

The final step in the process to collect balances due from a patient is to turn the account over to a collection agency and possibly dismiss the patient from the practice for nonpayment. Prior to using a collection agency, the facility should confirm that it has a current address for the patient and has been sending monthly bills to the patient with no response for a reasonable period of time, in the range of 6 months. Unfortunately, many account balances are written off or turned over to collection for something as simple as a transposition error on an address or the failure to send out account billings. The result can be financial losses to the facility or the loss of a valued patient who is upset about being pursued by a collection agency. After the facility has attempted unsuccessfully to collect the balance due, the sooner the collection agency receives the charge to collect, the better the results. Dismissing a patient from the practice is a serious step and should be backed by strong and clearly written financial policies.

Physician and Staff Training

The first step in a successful revenue cycle management program is the development of effective financial policies. With policies in place, the key to success lies in training, periodic reinforcement of policy, and workload management.

Case Study 11-2

Mrs. Johnson is an established patient of the medical practice. She comes into the office for her scheduled appointment and is seen by Dr. Smithers. At the checkout station, instead of paying her office visit copayment, she informs the cashier: "Dr. Smithers said that I did not have to pay today." The cashier reports the incident to the practice manager.

What steps should the practice manager take in a case like this?

Training and Follow-Up

All new employees and employees promoted or transferred to new positions need to be properly trained on revenue cycle management procedures. Periodically, the supervisor will need to reinforce the importance of financial policies with all employees of the medical facility, including the physicians, and will need to make sure that procedures are being properly followed. This review should include informal interviews with employees and reviews of documentation such as daily cash reports, reimbursement request forms, and accounts receivable aging reports.

Managing Workload

In any successful medical facility, increasing workload will lead to bottlenecks in the system. A single employee at the checkout may not be sufficient to both accept payments and schedule future appointments for patients. Personnel assigned to accounts receivable may not be able to handle all insurance billings and patient billings, and also make all of the accounting entries required to record payments received. Adding staffing should be the last alternative considered, not the first. The supervisor should review workload assignments of all staff members of the accounting function to determine if workload may be rebalanced among staff members. Training should be reviewed to ensure that all staff members are as efficient as possible in their daily work. The time savings of enhanced technology should also be explored.

Training the Patients

A critical component in revenue cycle management is getting patients to accept changes in financial policies. A practice that routinely collects no payments from patients until the insurance claim has been settled and the exact amount due from the patient is known will find it a challenge to have the patient pay estimated charges at time of service. Practices that have been lax in billing patients may encounter patient resistance when monthly bills are sent out and actions by collection agencies are threatened. Patients need to be treated professionally but firmly, stating the need for the improved financial policies and encouraging patient compliance.

Knowledge Check

11.1

1. Ann Reynolds has recently been hired as practice manager for Dr. LaRue. In reviewing the financial records of the practice, she notices that a substantial amount of money is owed by patients with outstanding balances. Further review finds that the practice has no written financial policies outlining the responsibility of patients in paying for their costs of medical care. Outline a set of basic financial policies to address patient responsibility for payment of charges.

_____

_____

_____

2. Tom Gregory is the practice manager for a local urologist. The practice has a detailed set of financial policies dealing with required payments from patients, but the staff have not been enforcing the policies and patients are not familiar with the requirements or the reasoning behind these policies. How does Mr. Gregory address this issue?

_____

_____

_____

Billings to Insurance Companies and Government Programs

As noted earlier, revenues from private-pay patients make up a very small percentage of the revenues of a medical facility. The great majority of the revenues come from reimbursements under contracts with healthcare insurance providers or from government programs. These claims are now filed electronically, and any minor error on the forms submitted will result in the claim being rejected and returned to the facility. This results in a time delay in reimbursement and staff costs for reworking the claim.

Best Practices to Accurately File Claims

The following are some best practices to enhance the accuracy of filing claims and timely reimbursement of funds due to the facility:

- Encounter form
- Coding changes
- Resident coding expert
- Reviewing charges in advance of submitting claims
- Billing errors
- Ensuring accurate reimbursements
- Negotiating insurance contracts

The Encounter Form

The encounter form is the basis for reimbursement of medical services in a physician's office. The form provides the specific information for the purposes of billing. It includes a selection of CPT codes for the provider to mark. A CPT code is a five-digit code used to identify the services provided. For example, it may be an office visit, a lab test, or an x-ray. In many instances, the basic encounter form is a standardized form that has been revised for the specific needs of the practice. The encounter form will also include the ICD-10-CM code or codes for the patient encounter that day. These codes provide diagnostic information about the patient. ICD-10-CM and CPT procedure codes may be included on the form for services that are rarely or never used by the practice. The form may be easily simplified by including only those codes for services routinely provided by the practice. Encounter forms should be numbered so that any missing forms may be tracked. With the implementation of the electronic health record, the encounter form is not always a piece of paper. For those practices where the billing system is integrated with the health record, the provider may be entering the information on the laptop as they complete the medical documentation by simply marking boxes on the screen.

Coding Changes

A computer-generated encounter form should be used to allow for quickly and easily revising the form as needed. Annually, the ICD-10 and CPT codes should be reviewed to delete codes for services not performed and to add codes for services currently being provided. Every year, codes are being revised and the current codes need to be included on the forms. Outdated codes will result in denied claims.

Resident Coding Expert

Every medical facility should have someone on-site who is trained and classified as their on-site coding expert. This person is responsible for implementing all coding changes and ensuring that all individuals involved in the revenue process are familiar with the changes.

Review of Charges in Advance of Submitting Claims

While the physician normally will complete and file the encounter form, a quality control process is essential to receiving full reimbursement for services. Depending on the type of medical facility, a medical assistant or nurse will be charged with the responsibility of ensuring that all medical services provided are accurately entered on the claim form. Documentation that is not complete or is not accurate will result in revenue losses to the facility. An error commonly made is to intentionally undercode for services provided to make sure that the facility is not accused of overcoding services. The solution is full and complete documentation and accurately coding for medical services provided.

Billing Errors

Errors in billing will happen, and the goal of revenue cycle management is to both reduce the number of errors and establish procedures to ensure that errors are fixed and claims resubmitted on a timely basis. A number of errors, such as inaccurate or expired insurance information and the lack of required precertification, cannot be fixed with rework, and those revenues are forever lost. The only action that can be taken is to strengthen procedures prior to medical service to compile correct information and obtain necessary precertifications. Many errors can be corrected with rework, and the claims resubmitted; however, the facility has had to dedicate extra staff time to the rework. A review of claims rejected will allow the facility to develop procedures to limit the number of future denials. An estimated one-third of all claims initially denied by insurance providers and governmental programs are never refiled, a huge revenue loss to the medical community.

Ensuring Accurate Reimbursements

Medical facilities will deal with a number of third-party insurance companies and government programs. In dealing with insurance companies, each will have a contract with the medical facility, outlining the terms and conditions of the contract and providing a schedule of reimbursements for medical services. The finance department or practice administrator should have easy access to the current contract from each company that the facility deals with. Insurance companies can make mistakes, and the facility should have a practice of periodically matching revenues actually received to the schedule of reimbursements. Insurance companies should also be monitored for the length of time it normally takes to receive reimbursement. If their turnaround time is not addressed in the contract, state law may provide prompt pay legislation.

Negotiating Insurance Contracts

Insurance contracts are legal agreements negotiated between the medical practice and the insurance company, detailing the specifics of the agreement and providing a reimbursement schedule for specific medical services provided to patients covered by that insurance program. The relationship between the medical facility and the insurance company should be a partnership in meeting the medical service needs of the members of the insurance program. Historically, the partnership has been one-way, with the insurance company dictating the terms of the contract and the amounts paid to reimburse the medical facility for services provided. A medical facility, as in any other line of business, needs to cover costs and make a reasonable profit to stay in business and continue to meet the service needs of the patients. In negotiating a contract with an insurance company, the facility needs to know their costs and what the insurance company proposes to reimburse.

Medical Facility Average Cost

The first step in the process of analyzing the profitability of a medical facility is to take the total operating costs of the medical facility for a period of time and divide that total by the number of patients seen during that period of time. Annualized numbers are best, but 3- or 6-month data may be used if the medical facility does not experience major seasonal fluctuations. The result is the **medical facility average cost**, or the average cost to see one patient. This cost number should be multiplied by a factor to provide for a reasonable profit margin.

Example 11-1

The practice administrator for a family medical practice uses operating expenses from last year's report from the outside accountant and divides by the total number of patients seen during that year. The resulting cost per patient is $83.65, and the medical facility feels that a profit margin of 30 percent is appropriate. $83.65 times 1.3 yields a required insurance reimbursement average of $108.75 to meet the goal of covering costs and providing a profit. Once this targeted average reimbursement has been determined, the next step in the process is to compare that cost figure with the average reimbursement rate paid by insurance contracts. To calculate the average reimbursement rate, determine the top 20–25 diagnosis codes used by the practice for medical service and average the reimbursement rates from the insurance company. The company needs to be reimbursing the medical facility at least $83.65 per patient visit to cover costs and at least $108.75 to provide the profit margin. If the proposed reimbursement rates in the contract will not provide the facility with those amounts, the practice needs to negotiate with the insurance company for higher reimbursements, using their actual cost figures as justification. When there is a single insurance company that covers a majority of the residents in the area, negotiation can be difficult, but the effort is still worthwhile.

This analysis is effective in instances where the medical facility is operating efficiently and the daily appointment book is consistently filled. When the medical facility is actively looking for new patients to fill the appointment book, the issue of **medical facility marginal cost** needs to be considered. Marginal costs are the additional costs incurred for the facility to see one additional patient. When additional patients or clients are able to be seen without increasing staff or using overtime, these marginal costs will be limited to the use of expendable medical supplies. Example 11-2 illustrates this.

Example 11-2

Southland Imaging Center saw a total of 4,000 patients last year, and total operating costs were $400,000, for a per-patient average visit cost of $100. This year, costs increased to $410,000, primarily from the use of additional medical supplies. Total patient visits increased to 4,400, reducing the per-patient average visit cost to $93.18. The reduction in the costs of an average visit will make it easier for the facility to cover expenses and provide a profit margin with the limited reimbursements allowed by insurance companies and government programs.

The insurance companies will also press medical facilities to accept their standard contract language for new contracts and for contract renewals. All provisions in the contract should be reviewed and any offensive sections negotiated. Common in these types of contracts are requirements on the number of days the facility has to submit a claim after providing medical services to a plan member, but no time limit is specified on the amount of time the company has to pay claims. The full contract needs to be reviewed carefully and discussed with the agent of the insurance company to ensure that the medical facility is treated fairly.

Electronic Claims Clearing Houses

The previous discussion dealt with medical facilities handling their own electronic claims billing. Several million medical professionals and businesses bill several thousand healthcare insurance companies located in all 50 states with a wide variety of state insurance regulations and software packages. These complexities have resulted in the creation of a new business model: the electronic claims clearing house.

A medical facility contracts with one of the dozens of regional clearing houses for a monthly fee based on the average volume of claims handled. The medical facility creates an electronic file of claims to be submitted and uploads the file to the contracted clearing house. The clearing house "scrubs" the claims (verifying the accuracy of the claims submitted) and electronically transmits the claims to the proper insurance companies. Errors on claims are caught quickly, and the claim is returned to the facility for corrections. Clearing houses have established relationships and secure connections with all major insurance companies. Claims are reviewed by the insurance company for accuracy and to ensure that the patient or client is currently insured. Insurance companies pay the individual medical facility electronically through the Automated Clearing House (ACH) banking system, and the facility is provided with an explanation of benefits (EOB).

Clearing houses include organizations that process nonstandard health information to conform to standards for data content or format, or vice versa, on behalf of other organizations.

Providers who submit HIPAA-like claims electronically are covered. These providers include but are not limited to:

- Doctors
- Clinics
- Psychologists
- Dentists
- Chiropractors
- Nursing homes
- Pharmacies

The services of the electronic claims clearing house are not free. A small medical facility that bills only one or two insurance carriers and has developed effective working relationships with those carriers may not need the service. A clearing house service may be an advantage to a facility billing multiple private-sector insurance companies and government programs and hindered by a small staff with limited expertise. Use of a clearing house is designed to catch billing errors more quickly, speed up the collection process, and allow all insurance claims to be submitted in one batch rather than being sorted by insurance provider.

Knowledge Check 11.2

1. Granite State Medical is experiencing claims denials in a larger percentage than industry average. As the practice administrator, what steps would you take to bring down the percentage of denials?

_____

_____

_____

2. As practice manager for a single-physician medical office, you notice that the physician is coding most patient contacts as simple office visits, and the practice is reimbursed by insurance at the lower reimbursement level. How do you ensure that the practice is paid for all appropriate costs of medical services provided?

_____

_____

_____

Revenue Losses in the System of Appointments

An established management principle is that work expands to meet the time available. An employee has 40 hours of work to be accomplished during the week and works diligently to have it completed. A second employee has work that can be finished in 20 to 25 hours per week but manages to look busy throughout the week. This same principle applies to the flow of patient care in a physician's office. On the surface, the practice may seem to be operating smoothly and efficiently, when there is actually time available to add additional appointments to the schedule without affecting patient care.

Using the example of the Southland Imaging Center from Example 11-2, the revenue from the average patient visit is $100. By taking steps to reduce missed appointments and scheduling some appointments for less time with the physician, the facility is able to see three additional patients per day. This does not sound like that much, but annual revenues would be increased by $75,000. All businesses are concerned about the bottom line, and $75,000 in new revenues with no major changes to the way the business operates should be sufficient to get attention.

There are finite limits to the number of patients that may be seen daily by the medical facility. When the facility manager sees only standing room in the waiting room, hears of patient complaints of long waits, and has employees and patients complaining of being rushed, the scheduling system may have been pushed a little too far. Maximizing revenues is always a balancing act between seeing as many patients as possible and providing the best possible medical care and convenience for the patients.

Timing of Appointments

Many physician practices have started to schedule some patient visits for as little as 10 minutes to be able to accommodate more patients during the workday. When effective, this both increases the revenue for the practice and allows patients to schedule visits without a lengthy delay to get an appointment. The following are guidelines used for the time scheduled for appointments:

- **10-minute short visit**: minor complaints, simple follow-up or check of medicines prescribed, established patients with a single symptom
- **20-minute standard visit**: new patients with a single symptom, established patients with multiple symptoms or chronic health problems
- **30-minute long visit**: new patients with chronic health problems, established patients with serious health issues, pre-employment physicals, and annual physical examinations

This type of scheduling can only be effective when all parties are involved in the process. The patient needs to understand the importance of being on time for the appointment, staff need to move the patients into examination rooms quickly and efficiently, and the physician needs to start on time and stay on time throughout the day.

Missed Appointments

Missed appointments pose a continuing problem for medical facilities. Staff need to be trained on treating patients politely but firmly, and patients need to be trained on the importance of meeting appointments. Each contact with the patient should reinforce this importance.

Figure 11-2 shows the cancellation rate based on how far out the appointment date is.

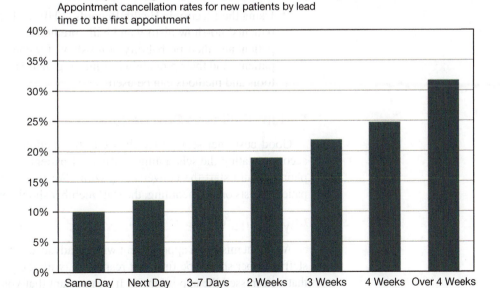

Figure 11-2 Cancellation Rates for First Appointments

Cancellation rates for first appointments, the data show, are closely correlated with how far out those appointments are scheduled. On average, a new patient who waits more than a month for a first appointment is more than twice as likely to cancel and not reschedule as a new patient who is scheduled within a week.
Source: athenahealth
Sample: 4.2 million appointments across 13,000 providers on the athenahealth network, for appointments scheduled in 2016. New patients are defined as patients who have not visited the practice in the last 3 years. Cancel rates are defined as the percent of new patient appointments cancelled and not rescheduled within six months of the original appointment.

Setting the Appointment

The patient calls to set an appointment. The staff member answering the phone finds an open time slot convenient for the patient. Most people now have both home and cell phones, and many of those employed will also have a work number. All phone numbers should be recorded and the patient asked which number is preferable for being contacted. The staff member should end the call by saying something like "We're reserving this time for you," stressing the point that it is important for the patient to meet the appointment. Care must be taken to comply with HIPAA patient privacy requirements in discussions with family members and in leaving phone messages.

Confirming the Appointment

It has been well documented that a confirming phone call the day prior to the appointment reduces the rate of missed appointments. People are busy and can easily forget an appointment. Many of these calls will go to voice mail and the staff member needs to be trained to leave a brief, concise message. This is another opportunity to stress the importance of meeting the appointment, by saying something such as "The doctor will be expecting you at 10 a.m. tomorrow," rather than "We hope to see you then."

There are a variety of strategies that can be used to verify the appointment. Using a variety of approaches can be beneficial to reaching various patients. Some strategies that can be used are:

- Shortening the waiting time between the scheduled and actual appointment. Patients tend to be sensitive to time delay, and any lead time higher than 2 weeks can significantly increase the probability of failing to attend the appointment.

- Adding automated reminders to adjust patient behaviors (text messages, phone calls, emails). Earlier studies showed a reduction of no-shows from 20.99 percent to 7.07 percent thanks to the telephone reminders.

- Establishing a separate cancellation phone line and using smart communication language in phone call reminders. These give the patient the comfort and the courage to cancel the booked appointments if they are no longer needed.

- Using the Electronic Health Records (EHRs). Healthcare providers can access patients' no-show history and build predictive models that can assess each patient and their probability of no-show. By considering the no-show record of patients and their probability of missing their appointment, predictive analytics tools and methods can be used.

Patient Calling to Reschedule

Good customer service requires that the medical office be reasonably flexible in accommodating the scheduling conflicts of patients. The staff members answering the phone should start the conversation with "We reserved this time for you." When the patient insists on rescheduling, the staff member should professionally honor the request.

Physician's Office Calling a Missed Appointment

A patient misses an appointment with no advance notice. When calling the patient, the staff member should be firm, but respectful, with the patient, saying "We're concerned that you missed the appointment. It's important that you see the doctor." For those few patients who continuously miss appointments, a face-to-face counseling session may be required.

Knowledge Check

11.3

1. John Donald is an established patient of the medical practice with chronic health conditions. Mr. Donald also has a history of missing appointments without any prior notification to the practice. As the practice manager for the office, what steps would you take to convince Mr. Donald to stop missing appointments?

_____

_____

_____

2. Drs. Findley and Rocker are partners in a family medicine practice. The practice appears to be busy and well run, but always seems to be short on cash at the end of the month. Billing rates are appropriate, and staff member salaries and draws of the partners are in line with the area. You are the practice administrator, and the partners have asked that you review the problem and make recommendations. What areas will you look at to improve the revenues of the practice?

_____

_____

_____

Key Concepts

- Revenue cycle management involves the collection of accounts receivable as quickly and completely as possible and requires the continuous attention of the financial management staff of any medical facility.

- Written financial policies, combined with training of staff, physicians, and patients, and workload management, are essential to the success of the revenue cycle management program.

- Management of the process of receiving funds owed by insurance and government programs includes a user-friendly encounter form, establishment of a position of in-house coding expert to stay current with coding changes and review charges for service for appropriate coding, and the review of billing errors to lower the percentage of claim denials.

- Revenues are lost both through the scheduling of appointments for the wrong amount of time and through missed appointments. Medical facilities can improve the bottom line by reviewing the process of scheduling appointments and in counseling patients on missed appointments.

Managing Financial Risk

Key Terms

Affirmative action

Age Discrimination in Employment Act (ADEA) of 1967

Americans with Disabilities Act (ADA) of 1990

Automobile liability insurance

Crime insurance

Directors and officers (D&O) liability insurance

Equal Employment Opportunity Commission (EEOC)

Equal Pay Act of 1963

Family and Medical Leave Act (FMLA) of 1993

General liability insurance

Insurance

Lilly Ledbetter Fair Pay Act of 2009

Litigation

Medical malpractice insurance

Occupational Safety and Health Administration (OSHA)

Pregnancy Discrimination Act (PDA) of 1978

continues

Chapter Objectives

After completing this chapter, readers should be able to:

- Explain basic components of the framework of risk management.

- Explain the financial impact of safety programs in the workplace.

- Identify major legislation imposing conditions on dealing with job applicants and employees.

- Describe the process of transferring financial risk to others through the purchase of insurance.

Key Terms

Property insurance
Protected classes
Quality management (QM)
Risk management
Sexual discrimination
Sexual harassment
Title VII, Civil Rights Act of 1964
Workers' compensation insurance

Chapter Glossary

Affirmative action is the process of developing procedures to ensure that individuals in protected classes (defined later in this list) have equal access to employment.

Age Discrimination in Employment Act (ADEA) of 1967 requires that workers over the age of 40 receive equal treatment in the workplace.

Americans with Disabilities Act (ADA) of 1990 protects the rights of people who are disabled in the workplace and requires "reasonable accommodation" for people with disabilities.

Automobile liability insurance protects against risk from loss in accidents involving vehicles owned by the business.

Crime insurance protects against risks from loss of money and securities, such as employee embezzlement.

Directors and officers (D&O) insurance protects against risks involving actions of directors and officers of the business.

Equal Employment Opportunity Commission (EEOC) was created by Title VII of the Civil Rights Act of 1964 to enforce actions on discrimination in the hiring process.

Equal Pay Act of 1963 established the standard that similar wages must be paid for similar work.

Family and Medical Leave Act (FMLA) of 1993 provides a guarantee of continuation of employment after up to 12 weeks away from the job for family or medical issues.

General liability insurance protects against risks from common occurrences such as slip and fall.

Insurance protects businesses, individuals, or groups from the risks of financial loss. Premium payments for the transfer of risk are pooled with a large group of participants.

Lilly Ledbetter Fair Pay Act of 2009 amended the filing deadlines under Title VII of the Civil Rights Act of 1964.

Litigation is the process of taking a legal proceeding through the courts.

Medical malpractice insurance protects against risks of loss from the actions of medical professionals.

Occupational Safety and Health Administration (OSHA) is the federal agency that provides protections for employee safety in the workplace.

Pregnancy Discrimination Act (PDA) of 1978 requires that pregnancy be treated the same as any other medical or personal leave.

Property insurance protects against risks to property owned by the business from exposures such as fire and natural disasters.

Protected classes are members of recognized minorities, women, individuals over age 40, disabled persons, and individuals with special religious beliefs.

Quality management (QM) is the growing profession dedicated to excellence in service delivery.

Risk management is the organized process to identify, evaluate, reduce or eliminate, and transfer to others the costs of risks to patients, visitors, and the organization's staff and assets.

Sexual discrimination is covered under the U.S. Equal Employment Opportunity Commission's (EEOC) extended Title VII of the Civil Rights Act of 1964 prohibiting discrimination on the basis of sexual orientation and gender identity. Sexual discrimination under Title VII also covers discrimination based on pregnancy, childbirth, or a related medical condition. This protection extends to prevent the employer from determining when the employee should take time off based on their pregnancy.

Sexual harassment results from unwelcome sexual advances, physical contact that creates a hostile environment, or requests for sexual favors.

Title VII, Civil Rights Act of 1964 was the first major piece of legislation to prohibit discrimination in the hiring process.

Workers' compensation insurance provides medical treatment and continuation of income for employees injured on the job.

Introduction

All organizations, not just healthcare, face a variety of risks in doing business. In no particular order, a partial listing of these risks would include:

- Fire
- Natural disasters (tornadoes, hurricanes)
- Vehicle accidents
- Workers' compensation claims
- Violations of EEOC, ADA, or FMLA
- Theft
- Embezzlement of company funds
- Employee sabotage
- Professional negligence
- Product liability
- Slips and falls

While the preceding risks are common to many types of organizations, health care faces risks unique to the industry. Medical malpractice is the most common and most expensive of these. However, risks to the healthcare provider are also found in areas such as implied consent and the confidentiality of medical records. Errors in providing healthcare are also likely to have more serious implications than those found in other businesses. A consumer purchases an electrical appliance, takes it home, and finds it does not work as advertised. The manufacturer, through the distributor, will be responsible for the cost of replacing the product. A surgical error made by a physician or a nurse's mistake in providing medication to a patient may well result in serious injury or death and a much more expensive financial risk to the organization.

We live in an increasingly litigious society, and the dramatic increase in **litigation** has led to the rise of modern risk management to protect the financial integrity of the organization. Litigation is defined as the process of taking a legal proceeding through the courts. In healthcare, most litigation is in the form of a civil legal action, as opposed to a criminal action. A civil action is referred to as a tort, a wrongful act that results in the injury to someone's person, reputation, or property. An example of a tort would be an individual bringing a legal action against their physician for malpractice.

One of the ways torts are split up is by the mental state of the person who commits the wrongdoing; for example, torts often are caused by someone's negligence. When the person who acts wrongly actually intended to perform the action, it becomes what is known as an "intentional tort."

The three most common intentional torts are battery, assault, and false imprisonment.

Battery is defined as intentional, harmful, or offensive touching with the intent to do harm.

Assault is defined as causing someone to fear harmful or offensive touching.

False imprisonment is restricting someone from moving against their will.

In larger organizations, including healthcare, professionally trained risk managers and safety officers will head a team dedicated to the control of the various risks faced on a daily basis. The risk management officers will conduct safety inspections, review incident reports for trends, make recommendation for procedural changes, and provide employee training in areas of safety and controlling risks. In smaller medical practices, the practice manager will most likely be in charge of risk management and safety. Risk assessment will be much more informal with the office manager visually observing staff compliance with established procedures, providing coaching and training where appropriate. The practice manager will also need to have a basic understanding of federal laws in the area of employment and discrimination in the workplace. In these areas, ignorance of the law is definitely not an acceptable excuse, and shortcomings may lead to severe financial penalties.

Risk management for all healthcare organizations is a process dedicated to protecting the financial assets of the institution. Even in an organization fortunate enough to not have any legal claims, the costs of risk are high. Many larger healthcare facilities will employ a safety officer and make a substantial investment in staff safety training and facility improvements to make a safer workplace. Insurance premiums are a significant area of expense, and there are other related costs such as human resources expenses in policy development and training to meet federal mandates in employment. With the exposures and costs involved in managing risk, the board of directors of the organization need to have an understanding of the risk management program. Healthcare facilities will commonly have a comprehensive insurance program with an annual renewal. Approval of the annual renewal premiums provides a timely opportunity to update the board of directors on risk management activities.

The Framework of Risk Management

The process of managing risk is based on the techniques and procedures that the organization can use to minimize the risk of liability and, when a problem occurs, to minimize the impact. Effective risk management is designed to answer the following questions:

- What can go wrong?
- How will the organization respond if something does go wrong?
- If a financial loss results from a risk management issue, how will the bills be paid?

The following steps outline the risk management process:

- Identification of risk
- Evaluation of risk
- Reduction and elimination of risk
- Transfer of risk

Identification of Risk

The most time-proven method of risk identification is the review of incidents. In healthcare, incident reports will be required for medical mistakes, patient falls, and employees injured by sharps on the job. A large urban hospital has adopted a formal incident report and requires that they be used whenever an incident occurs. A separate incident report is prepared by each eyewitness to an incident, and the incident reports are submitted to the risk management office. Risk management establishes a file for each incident; this file includes a copy of the patient medical record when the incident affects a patient. In addition to the records management process designed to assist the organization in the event of litigation, risk management tracks incidents by type over time to develop trends. Items placed in the incident file must be screened by the risk manager with the understanding that the file may well be subject to disclosure in litigation.

This identification process is also used for nonmedical risks. The risk manager also reviews such areas as accounting procedures in place to safeguard against embezzlement of funds, inventory control procedures, the need for defensive driving training for employees routinely using company vehicles, and the proper storage and use of flammable materials.

Equally as valuable as the internal identification of risk is the information available to the risk manager from professional organizations and their publications. A single hospital in Florida had the experience of amputating the wrong foot of one patient and operating on the wrong knee of another. These unfortunate incidents served as a wake-up call that procedures prior to surgery needed to be strengthened. Facility staff will now commonly confirm and reconfirm with the patient and the medical chart which body part is to be operated on. If the right knee is to be operated on, the left knee is clearly marked "NO." Write-ups in trade magazines and discussions at professional seminars serve to alert risk managers in the industry to review the procedures in place in their own healthcare organizations, avoiding costly litigation and related damage to the reputation of the facility.

Evaluation of Risk

In the identification of risk, discussed earlier, raw data on the risks to the organization are developed from incident reports, safety inspections, and ongoing communication with frontline supervisors. These data are analyzed by the risk manager and areas of exposure to risk outlined. A determination is made on the severity of the risk encountered. As an example, a small rural hospital has identified two areas of risk: the safeguarding of the office's petty cash fund and lack of proper training of medical assistants in sterilization of equipment. Of the two, the loss of petty cash would have a minimal impact on the organization, whereas errors in sterilization may result in serious injury to patients and damage to the reputation of the hospital.

Reduction and Elimination of Risk

Risk managers can have a significant impact on the organization in their response to risks identified and evaluated. The goals of an effective risk management program can be summarized as:

- Reduce the number of preventable incidents to staff, visitors, patients, the facility, and its assets.

- Reduce the chance of lawsuits being filed from incidents.

- When claims are filed, minimize final costs of the claims.

Best practice procedures are recommended in areas where weaknesses, such as safety procedures to protect staff, visitors, and patients, have been noted. "Best practices" has become an industry buzzword. They refer to industry-specific processes that have become generally accepted and standardized over time as reliable ways to improve business operations. Trade groups for a specific industry will gather information on effective operating procedures from their members and distribute this information in conferences, seminars, and publications. An Internet search for "best medical practices" will provide extensive information on best practices for medical facilities.

Best practices are put in place using enhanced staff training, either conducted internally or with outside resources. More stringent controls over accounting operations and inventory are established. Safety in the workplace is stressed. Additional emphasis is placed on patient relations, proven to be effective in reducing the incidence of litigation. Each of these actions can serve to reduce the risk to the healthcare organization.

Example 12-1

A patient at a medical facility slips on a wet floor in the waiting room and sprains her ankle. The office manager or another staff member immediately comforts the patient and asks a medical assistant to place an ice pack on the ankle. The following day, the office manager calls the patient, asks how the ankle is feeling, and offers any needed assistance. Continued communication and offers to reimburse any patient costs as a result of the incident will tend to mitigate the potential for litigation.

The healthcare organization's top management team and, ultimately, the board of directors must be active participants in this process of reducing risk. Change commonly does not come easily; the endorsement of top management is essential for the success of the changes proposed. Often, the best practice procedures and enhanced training recommended will require the investment of funds, again requiring the support of top management. The responsibility of the risk manager is to outline the costs and benefits of the changes to the organization.

Transfer of Risk

The most common method of transferring financial risk is the purchase of **insurance**. Insurance programs are designed to protect against catastrophic losses to the organization that could impact its ability to continue as a going concern: severe fire damage to a hospital, a major malpractice jury award, or the loss of large amounts of money from embezzlement. Annual premiums for insurance will be negotiated based on the total amount of coverage required and the degree to which the healthcare facility will participate in the risk, depending on the size of the deductible or the level of self-insurance required by the plan. An individual with a good driving record will be able to negotiate a lower premium for car insurance than an individual with a lengthy record of moving violations and accidents. Likewise, the loss experience of the organization will significantly impact premiums required for coverage.

Insurance may be obtained from traditional insurance carriers or through an insurance pool, where similar organizations agree to share in losses, essentially spreading the risk over a much larger base. Medical facilities will frequently use an insurance consultant to assist in purchasing insurance, both in determining the types and amount of coverage needed and in negotiating premiums. The insurance consultant will assist in ensuring that there are no gaps in coverage.

Knowledge Check

12.1

1. What is the first step in the risk management process?
   A. Transfer of risk
   B. Reduction and elimination of risk
   C. Evaluation of risk
   D. Identification of risk

2. What is the purpose and function of the use of an outside consultant in the risk management process?

_____

_____

_____

continued

3. A healthcare facility starts an aggressive program to reduce risks. After 2 years, the facility sees a marked reduction in incidents. The facility should see:

A. An increase in insurance premiums

B. A reduction in insurance premiums

C. No change in insurance premiums

Maintaining a Safe Work Environment

The safety of the physicians, staff, patients, and visitors is a critical part of the risk management and safety function of any healthcare facility. Providing a physically safe environment not only makes common sense, it makes good business sense. All facilities should have appropriate measures in place to protect the patients and staff.

BOX 12-1 Standard Precautions

Standard precautions, available from the Centers for Disease Control and Prevention, are a good starting point for developing safety policies:

1. Wear gloves to prevent the exposure of skin and mucous membranes to potentially infectious materials, including blood.

2. Remove and discard gloves immediately after finishing a procedure; avoid touching anything another person might touch without gloves.

3. Make point-of-use disposal units widely available to prevent sharps injuries.

4. Use gowns and aprons to prevent the anticipated soiling of clothing by blood or body fluids.

5. Wash hands before and after any contact with patients.

6. Use goggles and masks in procedures involving splashes or droplets.

Source: U.S. Department of Health and Human Services, Public Health Service, Centers for Disease Control & Prevention. (1993). *Guidelines for Prevention of Transmission of Human Immunodeficiency Virus and Hepatitis B Virus to Health Care and Public Safety Workers* (No. 550-17/80031). Washington, D.C.: Government Printing Office.

Occupational Safety and Health Administration (OSHA)

The **Occupational Safety and Health Administration (OSHA)** (www.osha.gov) is the federal agency that works to prevent injuries and protect the safety of the American workplace.

In 2019, U.S. hospitals recorded 221,400 work-related injuries and illnesses, a rate of 5.5 work-related injuries and illnesses for every 100 full-time employees. This is almost twice the rate for private industry as a whole.

OSHA is part of the U.S. Department of Labor, but OSHA staff work closely with the individual states in establishing guidelines and standards to promote worker safety and health.

For private industry and local government hospitals, which are predominantly medical and surgical hospitals, the most common event leading to injuries in 2015 was overexertion and bodily reaction, which included injuries from lifting or moving patients.

This event accounted for 45 percent of cases (24,040) in private hospitals and 44 percent of cases (3,090) in local government hospitals. The second most common event leading to workplace injuries and illnesses in private industry and local government hospitals was falls, slips, and trips. This event represented 25 percent of cases (13,230) in private hospitals and 24 percent of cases (1,690) in local government hospitals.

OSHA issues general guidelines, and each state has additional guidelines in the area of office safety. All employers, regardless of the size of the organization, are required to follow OSHA standards. Medical and dental offices are currently exempt from maintaining an official log of reportable injuries and illness under federal OSHA record-keeping rules; however, some states may require such record keeping.

Workers' Compensation

Workers' compensation insurance provides protection for employees injured on the job and is required by law in all states. The program includes payments for the treatment and rehabilitation of the employee and compensation until such time as the employee has been medically cleared to return to work. Each employer is assessed a premium based on the number of employees, payroll size, and a factor to account for the degree of danger of injury associated with specific occupations. The rating factor for an office worker will be low; the rating factor for a firefighter will be high. Each employer is assigned a modification factor that will increase or reduce the premium, based on that employer's claims history.

Since workers' compensation is regulated by law in individual states, claims brought under the law are handled by state courts under legal provisions that vary from state to state. Legal precedents from these cases apply only in the state where the judgment has been made. States have taken steps to combat the growing volume of lawsuits based on employee injury. As examples:

- The State of Florida has attacked the problem of growing lawsuits by statutorily limiting attorney fees in workers' compensation cases.

- The State of Washington approved sweeping changes to workers' compensation in 2011, designed to save millions of dollars in program expenditures.

Enhancing safety in the workplace and improving positive outcomes of medical procedures have an obvious beneficial impact on every healthcare organization.

There are several ways to help control workers' compensation costs.

1. Having a positive experience was associated with self-reported return to work. It suggests that speeding up claims and making them easier can help get employees back to work faster, which in turn lowers the costs of claims due to short periods of lost time.

2. Researchers found that nurse case management and early nurse referral can result in an average savings of $6,000 to $26,000 by ensuring workers get the best care and can return to work quickly. The results found that engaging nurses early could knock as much as 50 percent off the medical bill.

3. When an insurer accepts a claim upon application, it pays an average of $10,153. A denied-to-approved converted claim costs $15,694.

Working toward those ends is the goal of the growing field of **quality management (QM)**. QM, sometimes titled **quality improvement (QI),** is a process that has grown in stature over the past several decades. QM is a mechanism to formalize the investigation of critical areas within the organization. It is a collaborative effort between the administrative staff of the medical facility and the medical professionals, designed to quickly identify problem areas and take steps for appropriate corrective action. QM has evolved to the point where it is now a recognized specialty within healthcare with its own best practices and professional training for practitioners.

Knowledge
Check

12.2

1. Patricia Summers is a registered nurse employed at Smithville Community Hospital. During her work shift, she slips on a wet spot on the floor and severely twists her knee. She is out of work for 2 weeks recuperating from the injury. Which of the following insurance policies covers her medical costs and lost wages?

A. Medical malpractice insurance

B. Workers' compensation insurance

C. General liability insurance

D. Property insurance

2. The nursing manager at Smithville Community completes an incident report on the nurse injured by a fall caused by a wet spot on the floor. What safety policy should have been in place or should have been enforced to eliminate this dangerous condition?

_____

_____

_____

3. Why is workers' compensation insurance required in all states?

_____

_____

_____

Legal Issues in the Workplace

A complex and growing body of law is determining the rights of employees in the workplace. This section provides a brief overview of the more important employment regulations and is not designed to replace specialized courses on this subject available in many curricula.

Case Study 12-1

Aria Bowen is the practice manager for a smaller medical practice with two physicians and support staff. She started with the practice as a medical assistant and was promoted to practice manager a little over a year ago. She has developed competency in the bookkeeping functions of the practice and has begun to take classes online in a degree program for healthcare administration. Ms. Bowen is familiar with the pay structure in other healthcare facilities in the area and has noticed that their pay is falling behind others. With the approval of the partners, she has implemented a program that will provide a 10 percent raise to each employee, on their anniversary date of employment, based on a satisfactory performance review.

continued

The support staff in the practice generally work well together with the exception of two medical assistants who have an obvious personality clash. One of these staff members, Iris Brymer, comes into Ms. Bowen's office and says: "You just gave Adam Snelling a raise, and he now makes more than I do. We do the same work, and I have been here longer than Adam. If you don't fix this, I will hire a lawyer and sue you."

What is the appropriate action for Ms. Bowen to take on this issue?

Over the past half century, a growing body of law has evolved to protect the rights of individuals, from the application and selection process through their rights in the workplace. In larger organizations, the human resources department will be well versed on these laws and will train supervisors and employees of their rights and responsibilities. As with other issues, this burden will fall to the practice manager in smaller healthcare facilities. In addition to the ethical responsibilities of treating all employees fairly, violations of these laws can prove to be expensive and damaging to the organization.

The broad concept of these laws is that each individual should be treated equally in all employment issues, having an equal opportunity for employment regardless of age, race, gender, disabilities, or religion and then to be treated fairly and equally after employment.

Title VII, Civil Rights Act of 1964

Title VII, Civil Rights Act of 1964 was the first major piece of legislation to address discrimination in the hiring process. The act created the **Equal Employment Opportunity Commission (EEOC)** to enforce Title VII. Record keeping is required of employers with as small a workforce as 15 employees.

Members of recognized minorities, women, all individuals over 40, individuals with disabilities, and those with special religious beliefs are considered to be members of **protected classes**. **Affirmative action** is the process of developing procedures to ensure that individuals in these protected classes are afforded equal access to employment.

The act, together with interpretations provided by court cases, has resulted in a clearly defined list of dos and don'ts for questions that may be asked of job applicants. Some of these are obvious, others less so. The following are examples of questions that are prohibited under the act:

"Are you married?"

"How many children do you have?"

"In what year were you born?"

"What church do you attend?"

"Did you receive an honorable discharge from the military?"

"Have you ever filed a workers' compensation claim?"

"You have such a pretty complexion. What nationality are you?"

"Are there any religious holidays that you would not be available to work?"

"Are you a member of any local clubs, such as the Elks or Masonic Lodge?"

The interviewer still can get important information from the job applicant through questions that are acceptable under the act. Examples of questions that may be asked are:

"Are you legally eligible for employment in the United States?"

"Do you have any physical limitations that would affect your performance of job tasks outlined in the job description?"

"What professional associations are you a member of?"

"The standard work schedule for this position is Monday through Friday, 8 a.m. to 5 p.m. Would you find that schedule acceptable?"

Title VII Landmark Cases

The passage of Title VII started a lengthy period of litigation over the implementation of affirmative action and resulted in a number of landmark decisions from the U.S. Supreme Court:

- 1971: **Griggs v. Duke Power Co.** (401 U.S. 424). Employment practices that have a discriminatory impact are prohibited, even when those practices were not intended to be discriminatory.

- 1978: **Regents of the University of California v. Bakke** (438 U.S. 265). The admissions policy of the university was invalidated by the court; however, minority preferences were held to be acceptable.

- 1979: **United Steelworkers of America v. Weber** (443 U.S. 193). Kaiser Chemical Corporation enacted an affirmative action policy that gave 50 percent of skilled jobs to African Americans until the plant's racial makeup was the same as the community. The court upheld the policy.

- 1984: **Firefighters Local Union No. 1784 v. Stotts** (467 U.S. 561). The court ruled that a consent order authorizing the layoff of white firefighters to increase the percentage of minority firefighters was not enforceable.

- 1986: **Wygant v. Jackson (MI) Board of Education** (476 U.S. 267). A labor agreement between the union and the board of education, providing that white teachers with more seniority would be laid off prior to minority teachers with less seniority, was struck down by the court.

In a more recent U.S. Supreme Court action, the court agreed to hear two companion items coming from affirmative action cases involving the University of Michigan admissions policies. The two 2003 cases were **Gratz v. Bollinger** (539 U.S. 244) and **Grutter v. Bollinger** (539 U.S. 306). In 1995, Gratz, a white woman, applied for admittance into the university's undergraduate program. In 1997, Grutter, another white woman, applied for admittance into the university's law school. Both applications were rejected by the university. In the **Gratz** case, the undergraduate admissions policy was struck down by the court due to the fact that the admissions policy assigned a specific point value weighting to race in determining admissions. In the **Grutter** case, the law school admissions policy was allowed to stand. The law school policy used race as a criterion for admissions but did not assign a specific point value.

Affirmative action continues to be a work in progress:

> "A challenge from a white student who was denied admission to the University of Texas will be the high court's first look at affirmative action in higher education since its 2003 decision endorsing the use of race as a factor."
>
> *Mark Sherman, Associated Press, February 22, 2012*

The University of Texas admits most incoming freshmen from the top 10 percent of high school graduating classes. For the balance of new students admitted, race and other criteria are considered in granting admission. Abigail Fisher was not in the top 10 percent of her high school graduating class. She claims that minority students who were also not in the top 10 percent of their graduating classes were admitted when she was not, in spite of her superior academic record. The U.S. Supreme Court agreed to hear this case in the fall of 2012.

Sex discrimination under Title VII of the Civil Rights Act of 1964 also covers discrimination based on pregnancy, childbirth, or a related medical condition. This protection extends to prevent the employer from determining when the employee should take time off based on their pregnancy. If the employee is temporarily unable to perform all the duties of their job, the employer must offer the same accommodations that would be provided to a worker who was on short-term disability. This also extends to healthcare benefits that an employer must cover for employees.

The issue of **sexual harassment** is particularly troublesome in the healthcare setting. Sexual harassment results from unwelcome sexual advances, physical contact that creates a hostile environment, or requests for sexual favors. Most case law on sexual harassment arises from employment situations. In healthcare, sexual harassment includes inappropriate actions of a sexual nature from the medical staff toward patients or clients.

Sexual harassment is part of the broader subject of **sexual discrimination**. Although federal law does not explicitly prohibit employment discrimination based on "gender identity" or "gender expression," recent interpretations in case law under Title VII extend the Act's prohibition of sex discrimination to include bias based on gender identity and gender expression.

Bodily functions and patient sexual activity are legitimate discussions in healthcare as long as they are handled in a professional manner. Sex discrimination, including sexual harassment, is prohibited by Title VII. It is the responsibility of management to create a work environment free of sexual harassment and to stress to all employees that offensive activity will not be tolerated.

The Equal Pay Act of 1963

The **Equal Pay Act of 1963** requires that similar wages must be paid for similar work. For example, two new nurses were hired by a hospital with comparable education and experience. It would not be legal for the hospital to pay different starting wages if one nurse was male and the other female. The issue of **comparable worth** also comes into play in pay issues. Comparable worth states that if two jobs require comparable skills, knowledge, and abilities, even if the jobs are very dissimilar, the pay of the two positions should be similar. Comparable worth is the basis of professional classification and compensation plans.

The Age Discrimination in Employment Act (ADEA) of 1967

The **Age Discrimination in Employment Act (ADEA) of 1967**, including later amendments, established that workers over 40 are members of a protected class. All employers with 20 or more employees are required to comply with the act. Rights for older workers were expanded with the **Older Workers Benefit Protection Act of 1990**, requiring that older workers receive equal treatment when an organization is downsizing with offers of early retirement or enhanced severance packages.

Pregnancy Discrimination Act (PDA) of 1978

Any employer with more than 15 employees must treat pregnancy the same as any other medical or personal leave under the **Pregnancy Discrimination Act (PDA) of 1978**.

Family and Medical Leave Act (FMLA) of 1993

This law expanded the rights granted by PDA to provide leave rights for all employees. Under the **Family and Medical Leave Act (FMLA) of 1993**, all employees have the right to up to 12 weeks of family leave without pay, including the right to return to their same position or to an equivalent position with no loss in pay, benefits, status, or other terms and conditions of employment.

A major legal issue in FMLA has been the coordination between sick and personal leave by an employee and benefits afforded under FMLA. Employees would use their sick or personal leave to handle a "minor illness," while a "serious health condition" falls under FMLA. In **Caldwell v. Holland of Texas** (8th Cir. 2000, 208 F. 3d 671), an employee was terminated for excess absence treating the ear infection of her 3-year-old child. The court ruled that Caldwell was able to demonstrate that the ear infection was serious enough to impact the child's normal activities and that the benefits under FMLA should have been provided to the mother. In another case of termination for excess absence, a mother took time off to assist in the case of an adult daughter with asthma. In **Sakellarion v. Judge & Dolph Ltd.** (N.D. Ill. 1995, 893 F. Supp. 800), the court ruled that the daughter was capable of helping herself with the asthma and that FMLA did not apply.

The Americans with Disabilities Act (ADA) of 1990

The **Americans with Disabilities Act (ADA) of 1990** requires that any individual who can perform the essential tasks of a position cannot be discriminated against, and employers are mandated to make **reasonable accommodation** for individuals with disabilities, except when accommodation would cause **undue hardship** on the employer. These terms continue to be the subject of litigation. Additionally, pre-employment physicals are prohibited, except when combined with a conditional job offer. The employer must show essential job functions in a written job description, including the amount of time spent on each function and the importance of each.

The world of televised golf provided a well-publicized case study on ADA. Casey Martin was a professional golfer with a disability that would not allow him to walk the distances on a golf course. He appealed to the PGA Tour for an exemption to use a golf cart while all other competitors were required to walk. The PGA refused to provide him the exception. In **PGA Tour Inc. v. Martin** (532 U.S. 661 2001, S.Ct. 1879), the court ruled that Martin's disability fell under the provisions of ADA and he was entitled to use a golf cart.

Lilly Ledbetter Fair Pay Act of 2009

Employment law and the related financial exposures for businesses continue to evolve. The first act signed into law by President Obama, on January 29, 2009, was the **Lilly Ledbetter Fair Pay Act of 2009**. Ledbetter was a supervisor at a Goodyear tire plant who filed an equal-pay lawsuit under Title VII of the Civil Rights Act of 1964, claiming pay discrimination. The case was heard by the U.S. Supreme Court in **Ledbetter v. Goodyear Tire & Rubber Co.** (550 U.S. 618). The court ruled 5–4 that she had filed the claim too late to comply with the 180-day filing requirement in Title VII. The court's minority position was that any paycheck received that was found to be in violation restarted the 180-day clock. The Ledbetter Act was based on the minority position of the court and states that the 180-day filing requirement in Title VII starts anew with each discriminatory paycheck.

Knowledge Check 12.3

1. In Case Study 12-1 at the beginning of this section, the practice manager is faced with the situation where two employees, doing the same work, are paid at different rates of pay. What is the proper response to the upset employee?

_____

_____

_____

2. Federal legislation creating affirmative action and defining protected classes first appeared in which of the following acts?
   A. Family and Medical Leave Act of 1993
   B. Title VII, Civil Rights Act of 1964
   C. Health Insurance Portability and Accountability Act of 1996
   D. Americans with Disabilities Act of 1990

continued

3. Carol Fisher is employed in the medical records office of a local hospital. She was severely injured in a car accident and now uses a wheelchair because she is unable to walk. Which of the following federal acts requires "reasonable accommodation" in employment?

A. Family and Medical Leave Act of 1993

B. Title VII, Civil Rights Act of 1964

C. Health Insurance Portability and Accountability Act of 1996

D. Americans with Disabilities Act of 1990

E. None of the above

4. Under federal law, employees are guaranteed up to 12 weeks' leave for personal issues and family health problems with their jobs held for them. Which of the following federal acts provides this guarantee?

A. Family and Medical Leave Act of 1993

B. Title VII, Civil Rights Act of 1964

C. Health Insurance Portability and Accountability Act of 1996

D. Americans with Disabilities Act of 1990

E. None of the above

Financial Risk Transferred to Others

Each organization will have a number of areas of financial risk where those risks may be reduced through employee training and best-practice procedures, but never eliminated. These areas of financial risk may be transferred to others through the purchase of insurance. Specific areas of financial risk exposure that can be transferred by the purchase of insurance are property, general liability, and automobile liability.

Case Study 12-2

Dr. Asher Lee runs a single-practitioner family medical practice. Staffing for the practice includes Dr. Lee, a practice manager, and three medical assistants. Cora Robertson has served as the practice manager for a number of years, until her resignation before Thanksgiving to devote more time to family. Dr. Jones waited until after the holidays to interview and hire a new practice manager. Emma Johnson was hired as the new practice manager and started work in mid-February of this year. On her first day in the office, she found a sizable stack of correspondence that the medical assistants felt would be her responsibility. One letter, from American Surety & Casualty, notified her that the fire insurance policy covering business interruption and losses to the contents of the rented office space had been cancelled for nonpayment as of January 31. During a break in his patient load, Dr. Lee told Ms. Johnson that Ms. Robertson had handled everything related to the business side of the practice, but he thought a local insurance agent was used to arrange insurance.

What steps should Ms. Johnson take on the immediate issue of fire insurance? What further steps would be appropriate regarding the management of risk for the medical practice?

Property

The largest single item on the balance sheet of a healthcare organization is most likely to be the investment in real property and equipment. Even a single-physician medical office working out of leased office space will have a sizable investment in leasehold improvements and equipment. An "all perils" **property insurance** policy is preferable to a "named peril" policy in that the former removes the opportunity for disagreement on the cause of specific losses. Computer equipment will best be insured with an electronic data processing (EDP) rider to the property policy. Unusual items of property, normally of high value and difficult to replace quickly, will be described and appraised separately for insurance purposes. Specific items, such as property owned by others (normally leased equipment) and boiler and machinery, may also be covered by the property policy. "Boiler and machinery" requires a little explanation. Formerly, buildings were heated with steam heat with a boiler in the basement and radiators in each room. Because of the costs involved and the danger of boiler explosion, a separate policy for **boiler and machinery** coverage could be purchased. Today, this type of policy is purchased to insure specific pieces of expensive equipment.

General Liability

The **general liability insurance** policy will protect against issues arising from torts, a failure to act in a reasonable and prudent manner. Claims coming from this area of law will include hazards in the facility that cause damage or injury. A common example is a slip and fall claim filed by a visitor to the facility. Losses from tort claims can be expensive, including settlements for specific awards, such as medical expenses and loss of income; general awards, such as pain and suffering; and punitive awards, designed to punish reckless actions of the defendant.

Automobile Liability

Automobile liability insurance is statutorily required; a general auto policy will be sufficient when the healthcare facility only owns a few vehicles for use by top management and for facility maintenance and miscellaneous uses. Many large organizations will choose to self-insure the physical damage to their vehicles and only insure for liability. In areas where the local hospital also provides ambulance service, more attention must be given to proper liability and physical damage coverage.

Directors and Officers Liability

Hospitals, both for-profit and not-for-profit, will ask well-respected members of the community to serve on their board of directors. These individuals will expect that the healthcare organization will provide protection for their personal assets against lawsuits filed based on decisions made by the board of directors. **Directors and officers (D&O) liability insurance** will insure against claims for misuse of assets and errors and omissions of board members, as well as top executives of the organization, and may be expanded to cover other personnel involved in the administration of the facility.

Crime Insurance

A **crime insurance** policy may be a freestanding policy or written as part of the property insurance policy. Risks covered by this policy will include employee dishonesty, losses from robbery or theft both on and off premises, and losses from the illegal use of negotiable instruments (checks) of the organization.

Medical Malpractice

Medical malpractice insurance provides coverage for the financial risk to the medical facility resulting from errors in patient care. This is the largest area of risk in healthcare. The term **malpractice** in the healthcare setting refers to negligent actions of medical professionals such as physicians, nurses, and technicians. In addition to the individual professionals, medical malpractice may apply to healthcare institutions, such as hospitals. The term **negligent action** also requires definition. The commonly used definition is that negligence is the failure to exercise ordinary care. Through court cases, this has evolved into the "reasonable person" rule, holding that negligence occurs when the ordinary care that would be provided by a competent trained professional was not provided. Individual healthcare professionals and healthcare facilities face compensatory damage awards as a result of negligence, providing the patient with funds to cover loss of earnings as well as past and future medical costs directly arising from the negligence. Damage awards may also include awards for pain and suffering, loss of consortium, and mental anguish. Punitive damages may be awarded in cases of gross negligence. Medical malpractice insurance is available in the marketplace to protect the individual professional or institution from the financial risks of a large malpractice settlement. Insurance coverage for medical malpractice is very expensive, reflecting both the increasing volume of claims in this area and the high costs where negligence has been proven.

The purchase of insurance comes with technicalities that need to be understood to ensure that the facility has full coverage for claims. **Claims-made insurance** is a policy provision stating that only claims reported to the insurance company during the period of time that the policy is in force will be covered. A policy with a **claims-incurred** provision provides wider protection, covering claims made under the policy when the incident is within the dates that the policy was in force, regardless of the date of filing the claim with the insurance company. The danger of a claims-made policy comes when the healthcare facility is switching insurance to a different carrier. If an incident occurs during the old policy period, but is not reported prior to the policy expiring, neither the old nor the new insurance policy will provide coverage. To protect against this potential gap in coverage, the organization may choose to purchase **tail coverage** from the company providing the expiring insurance or **prior acts coverage** from the company writing the new policy. Both will provide protection in the case where the incident date was prior to the expiring insurance but not reported prior to the expiration date of the old policy.

Knowledge Check 12.4

1. In Case Study 12-2 at the beginning of this section, Cora Robertson is the new practice manager for a medical office. Correspondence received from the insurance company shows that insurance coverage has been cancelled for nonpayment. Outline the steps that Ms. Robertson should take, both to reinstate insurance coverage and to ensure that she is comfortable with the practice's risk management program.

_____

_____

_____

continued

2. The Northshore Medical Clinic is located in Madison, Wisconsin. Last February, Mr. Jenkins, a patient of the clinic, slipped on an icy sidewalk at the clinic, fell, and broke his hip. He brought a suit against Northshore, claiming negligence in not properly maintaining the sidewalk in winter conditions. Which of the following insurance policies will protect the finances of Northshore against potential losses from this suit?

   A. Medical malpractice insurance

   B. Directors and officers liability insurance

   C. General liability insurance

   D. Workers' compensation insurance

3. Sunrise Hospital serves a suburban community in the Phoenix, Arizona, area. Amelia Elder, president of the local bank, has been appointed to the hospital's board of directors. Sunrise is looking to expand facilities on their existing campus but is being sued by the adjacent residential neighborhood as being detrimental to their property values and quality of life. Sunrise and each of the individual members of the board of directors are named in the suit. Which of the following insurance policies protects Ms. Elder?

   A. Medical malpractice insurance

   B. Directors and officers liability insurance

   C. General liability insurance

   D. Workers' compensation insurance

   E. None of the above

4. Miguel Sanchez is employed in the food services department of a local hospital, responsible for receiving food orders and properly storing shipments in the hospital's inventory. In the process of moving heavy boxes, he severely strains his back and has to be off work for several weeks to recuperate. Which of the following insurance policies ensures payments of his medical expenses and provides continuation of income?

   A. Medical malpractice insurance

   B. Directors and officers liability insurance

   C. General liability insurance

   D. Workers' compensation insurance

   E. None of the above

5. Explain the difference between an insurance policy with a claims-made provision and a claims-incurred provision. What is the potential impact on the healthcare facility under these two options?

   _____

   _____

   _____

Key Concepts

- The process of risk management is important to safeguarding the finances of every healthcare organization. The process starts with identification of risks, the evaluation of these risks, actively working to reduce or eliminate risks, and the transfer of financial risks to others.

- A growing body of legislation has arisen over the past several decades protecting the rights of both job applicants and employees. All healthcare organizations need to understand these laws and ensure that the organization has taken steps necessary to ensure compliance. In smaller medical facilities without a human resources professional, these responsibilities fall to the practice manager.

- Healthcare professionals and facilities face risks that could be financially devastating. The transfer of these risks to others, through the purchase of insurance coverage, serves to protect the financial viability of the organization.

- Risk management, workplace safety, human resources, and quality management (QM) are each recognized professional careers within health care. This chapter has provided only a quick overview of the financial risks to the organization addressed by these professionals. Students with a desire to learn more on these issues are urged to take advantage of the many excellent professional associations and publications available.

Financial Management of Health Information Technology

Chapter

13

Chapter Objectives

After completing this chapter, readers should be able to:

- Define health information technology (HIT).

- Define a qualified electronic health record (EHR).

- Identify costs of adoption of ICD-10.

- Identify the impact of the coding structure.

- Describe how HIPAA impacts the business of health care.

- Explain how HIPAA protects a patient's right to privacy.

Chapter Glossary

The **American Recovery and Reinvestment Act of 2009 (ARRA)** was approved as a stimulus for capital investment. The act included funding for computerized medical records in a standardized format.

An **electronic health record (EHR)** is the health record of a patient kept in an electronic format by providers of medical service.

Electronic prescriptions (eRx) are an initiative of the federal government to have physicians use electronic means to send prescriptions to the patient and pharmacies.

Health information technology (HIT) is the hardware, software, integrated technologies or related licenses, intellectual property, upgrades, or packaged solutions sold as services that are maintenance, access, or exchange of health information.

Health Information Technology for Economic and Clinical Health Act (HITECH) of 2009 provided federal stimulus funding for the automation of healthcare records.

Health Insurance Portability and Accountability Act of 1996 (HIPAA) provides for the portability of healthcare benefits between employers, ensures the privacy of healthcare information, and requires the standardization of electronic healthcare communications.

The **International Classification of Diseases, Edition 10 (ICD-10-CM and ICD-10-PCS)** is a worldwide initiative for the improvement of medical diagnosis codes.

The **Medicare Improvements for Patients and Providers Act (MIPPA)** provides funding to agencies and organizations in all states or Native American tribes that are used for financial assistance to help eligible Medicare beneficiaries reduce their premiums and deductibles.

The **Medicare Modernization Act (MMA)** helped establish prescription drug coverage. It is viewed as a large benefit in Medicare history.

Introduction

Computer technology has redefined how we live, work, and play. The healthcare industry is no exception to this revolution. The major technological changes to be discussed are those that affect the business of health care, not the innovations and changes in clinical care. As defined by the American Recovery and Reinvestment Act of 2009 (ARRA), **health information technology (HIT)** is the hardware, software, integrated technologies or related licenses, intellectual property, upgrades, or packaged solutions sold as services that are designed for or support the use by healthcare entities or patients for the electronic creation, maintenance, access, or exchange of health information.

Since the adoption of the **Health Insurance Portability and Accountability Act of 1996 (HIPAA)**, the healthcare industry has been faced with a variety of new laws and regulations that affect the business of health care. Most people think of HIPAA as the reason for privacy protection in health care. Although HIPAA certainly does pertain to privacy, a variety of other changes that affected health information technology were also part of HIPAA. However, additional new laws were necessary to require the healthcare industry to move to the adoption of health information technology such as electronic medical records.

The first change came in 2008 when the **Medicare Improvements for Patients and Providers Act (MIPPA)** was passed. This legislation set up the **electronic prescription (eRx)** Incentive Program for providers who take care of Medicare patients. Although not directly related to HIPAA, this law provided incentives to physicians that use eRx for their patients who have Medicare.

Congress recognized the massive cost of converting manual medical records into a standardized automated format and approved the Health Information Technology for Economic and Clinical Health Act (HITECH) as part of the American Recovery and Reinvestment Act of 2009 (ARRA). This law provided monetary incentives but also required conversion to **electronic health record (EHR)**.

The Patient Protection and Affordable Care Act (PPACA) of 2010 requires the development of accountable care organizations for Medicare patients. This act requires a significant financial investment in infrastructure and technology to assist in high quality and efficient care.

Lastly, the implementation of the International Classification of Diseases Edition 10 (ICD-10-CM and ICD-10-PCS) in 2022 had a major impact on health information technology efforts.

ICD-10-CM/PCS has an improved structure, capacity, and flexibility for capturing advances in technology and medical knowledge. It incorporates greater clinical detail and level of specificity to provide better quality of data for many purposes. That greater clinical detail and specificity will also allow for more efficient tracking of healthcare and public health trends, quality of care issues, and evaluating health outcomes.

ICD-10 has benefitted providers with operational monitoring, research, accurate payments for new procedures, fewer miscoded reimbursement claims, a better understanding of the value of new procedures, and efficient disease management The benefits of ICD-10-CM and ICD-10-PCS impact new procedures, payments and improved disease engagement. These are shown in Table 13-1.

Table 13-1 Summary of Estimated Benefits over a Ten-Year Period

Category	Benefit ($ million)	Largely Due to
More-accurate payment for new procedures	100–1,200	ICD-10-PCS
Fewer rejected claims	200–2,500	both
Fewer fraudulent claims	100–1,000	both
Better understanding of new procedures	100–1,500	ICD-10-PCS
Improved disease management	200–1,500	ICD-10-CM

As the U.S. healthcare industry continues to advance both medically and technologically, a more modern coding structure is required to reflect and support these developments.

The new coding structure facilitates improvements in cost reduction, improve quality of care for patients, and update the way healthcare data are captured to positively affect health outcomes.

Health Insurance Portability and Accountability Act of 1996 (HIPAA)

The U.S. healthcare system has long recognized the need for privacy of an individual's medical records. However, this right to privacy lacked effective legislation for enforcement. HIPAA requires that all healthcare providers maintain rigorous standards to ensure that the privacy of the patient is protected.

Additionally, HIPAA requires portability of employee health insurance. These two parts of HIPAA are fairly well known to the general public. However, HIPAA had several other requirements for the healthcare industry. The accountability section of the act gave the healthcare industry three other specific standards to meet. They are:

1. Transactions and code sets: The act established a standard requiring the use of consistent billing and coding formats and data content when transmitting medical files electronically.

2. Security: When protected health information (PHI) is transmitted electronically, the act requires that the transmissions are done securely with password protection, firewalls, encryption, and antivirus software in place, as well as loss prevention.

3. National identifier: The act established a unique national identifier for medical service providers, health insurance plans, employers, and individuals.

Case Study 13-1

Riverside Medical Center is a community hospital providing for the medical needs of the local population. The community is fairly small with most townspeople knowing each other through school, business, or spiritual practices. Riverside prides itself on providing excellent medical care coupled with a caring attitude. Staff members have been trained to keep family and friends updated on each patient's progress when they call in for status reports. Patient names are clearly posted on doors so visitors can easily find the right room. With the passage of HIPAA in 1996, Riverside was forced to make significant changes to their patient privacy policies. Now with the implementation of EHR and ICD-10-CM, the medical center faces additional challenges.

Identify some of these challenges and possible solutions facing Riverside Medical Center.

Patients are covered by numerous insurance programs, some private and some governmental, each with their own individual forms and reimbursement requirements. A wide variety of computer programs are on the market to assist in records management and billing; however, these programs lack standardization and the ability to interface with each other. The electronic transactions were governed by the Accredited Standards Committee X12 Version 4010/4010A1 for healthcare transactions until December 31, 2011.

The U.S. Department of Health and Human Services (HHS) mandated that transaction standards for all electronic healthcare claims must be upgraded to Version 5010 from Version 4010/4010A by January 1, 2012. As of January 1, 2012, all **HIPAA**-covered entities must be compliant with Version 5010.

Version 5010 was designed to allow for successful conversion to ICD-10. The importance of ICD-10-CM will be discussed in a later section of this chapter. Box 13-1 lists covered entities under HIPAA. All covered entities must comply with 5010, as well as any other **HIPAA** rules.

BOX 13-1 HIPAA-Covered Entities

- Hospitals
- Physician practices
- Nursing homes
- Hospice care facilities
- Dentists
- Chiropractors
- Podiatrists
- Physical therapy centers
- Laboratories
- Medical clearinghouses
- Health insurance companies
- Alternative medicine providers

The issue of security for EHRs was addressed in the HIPAA legislation as well as ARRA. The ARRA increased the fines. All providers must address security threats from three different sources: human, environmental, and natural disasters. There must be administrative safeguards, as well as physical and technical safeguards. For example, electronic health information can be accessed through various methods within a healthcare system: at the front office, in an examination room, or on a mobile device. Healthcare professionals must be informed about practices used at the facility to safeguard patient information such as EHRs. Many healthcare facilities use mobile devices that access patients' EHRs. These mobile devices must be closely monitored to avoid a breach of patient information. Figures 13-1a, 13-1b, and 13-1c show examples of a location and devices used in healthcare facilities where patient information is accessed.

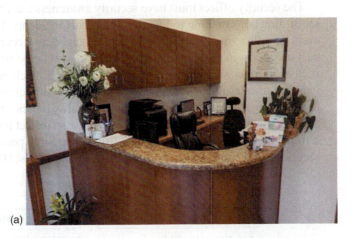

(a)

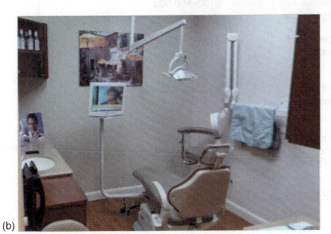

(b)

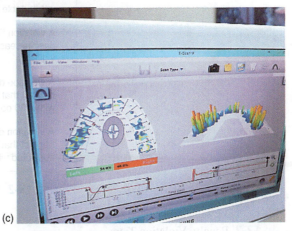

(c)

Figure 13-1 Healthcare Facilities Must have Practices in Place that all Employees Must Follow to Protect a Patient's Health Information and Avoid Violations and Penalties. These Practices Will Cover all Aspects of the Facility, Including (a) The Front Office, (b) Examination Rooms, and (c) Mobile Devices Used to Access a Patient's EHR.

The law now states that entities must self-report, and the fines and punishments can be steep. All covered entities must have developed both privacy and security practices that preserve patient confidentiality. The final rules from the federal government on privacy and security were released in 2012.

Between 2009 and 2021, 4,419 healthcare data breaches of 500 or more records have been reported to the HHS Office for Civil Rights. Those breaches have resulted in the loss, theft, exposure, or impermissible disclosure of 314,063,186 healthcare records.

Organizations will be expected to self-report any violation or face even stiffer penalties. Additionally, beginning in 2012, the federal government started unannounced audits of privacy and security processes in major healthcare facilities. HIPAA's security rule requires that an individual be designated to be in charge of the security program for the covered entity. This person is responsible for:

- Developing security goals and objectives

- Determining how the goals and objectives will be met

- Advising administration regarding information security

- Determining reporting procedures

- Conducting adequate risk assessment and determining the appropriate level of risk acceptance

The security officer must have security awareness training in place, as well as a clear set of directions on how to identify and report incidents. Plans must be in place in the event of a loss of data due to a system emergency. Records can be lost if there is no backup system in place. The possibility of loss could be from weather-related incidents such as hurricanes, tornadoes, or floods. However, hackers and other man-made problems can also result in a loss of data. The security officer must have plans to get the system working again and to update activity. Security policies and procedures must not only address how to prevent such loss of data, but also reflect how changes are made to keep it from happening again. Figure 13-2 lists the possible penalties for violation of HIPAA security and privacy rules, and Table 13-2 lists the latest HIPAA penalty violation tiers.

HIPAA VIOLATION	PENALTY
A violation of HIPAA attributable to ignorance	$100–$50,000
A violation that occurred despite reasonable vigilance	$1,000–$50,000
A violation due to willful neglect that is corrected within 30 days	$10,000–$50,000
A violation due to willful neglect that is not corrected within 30 days	$50,000

Figure 13-2 HIPAA Penalty Violations

Table 13-2 Penalty Violation Tiers

Penalty Tier	Culpability	Minimum Penalty per Violation – Inflation Adjusted	Max Penalty per Violation – Inflation Adjusted	Maximum Penalty per Year (cap) – Inflation Adjusted
Tier 1	Lack of Knowledge	$120	$60,226	$1,806,757
Tier 2	Reasonable Cause	$1,205	$60,226	$1,806,757
Tier 3	Willful Neglect	$12,045	$60,226	$1,806,757
Tier 4	Willful Neglect (not corrected within 30 days)	$60,226	$1,806,757	$1,806,757

Comprehension Check 13.1

In the following questions, list the minimum penalty based on the culpability.

1. Dr. Sergio hired a new dental assistant. The new assistant was not trained on how to close a patient's dental record. Based on the assistant's ignorance, what would be the minimum amount for the HIPAA violation?

2. Dr. Mangier was given a violation for an electronic breach based on discussing a patient's medical condition where patients in the waiting room could hear the conversation. She neglected to close the waiting room door when discussing the patient's information with her medical staff. What would be the minimum amount for the HIPAA violation?

3. Dr. Scitio had a power outage in the medical facility. As he was seeing a patient in one of the examining rooms, another patient's health record appeared on the computer monitor in the room. Even though Dr. Scitio explained to the patient it was a reasonable occurrence when the electricity goes off, the patient filed a complaint. What would be the minimum amount for the HIPAA violation?

The national provider identifier (NPI) is a unique identification number for covered healthcare providers. Covered healthcare providers, all health plans, and healthcare clearinghouses must use NPIs in the administrative and financial transactions adopted under HIPAA. The NPI is a 10-position, intelligence-free, numeric identifier (10-digit number). This means that the numbers do not carry other information about healthcare providers, such as the state in which they live or their medical specialty. This rule was fully adopted in 2008.

Knowledge Check 13.1

1. Riverside Chiropractic Center was forced to make changes to privacy policies as a result of HIPAA. What changes will need to be made for covered entities?

_____

_____

_____

2. A number of nursing homes have been fined for violations of the security of patient medical records under HIPAA. Research the Internet for examples of these violations and assessed fines.

_____

_____

_____

Medicare Improvements for Patients and Providers Act (MIPPA)

The Medicare Improvements for Patients and Providers Act (MIPPA) provides funding to agencies and organizations in all states or Native American tribes that are used for financial assistance to help eligible Medicare beneficiaries reduce their premiums and deductibles. Since its passage in 2008, MIPPA has helped more than one million low-income Medicare beneficiaries to access programs that make their healthcare and prescriptions costs more affordable. MIPPA grantees are located in all states, Puerto Rico, Guam, and the District of Columbia.

At the end of 2020, Congress passed and the President signed a large Omnibus spending package that included a 3-year extension of MIPPA through 2024. Annual funding for MIPPA outreach also increased from $37.5 million to $50 million with $15 million each for Area Agencies on Aging, State Health Insurance Assistance Programs, and the National Center for Benefits Outreach and Enrollment and $5 million for Aging and Disability Resource Centers.

Medicare Modernization Act (MMA)

The inclusion of electronic prescribing in the **Medicare Modernization Act (MMA)** of 2003 gave momentum to the movement, and the July 2006 Institute of Medicine report on the role of e-prescribing in reducing medication errors received widespread publicity, helping to build awareness of e-prescribing's role in enhancing patient safety. Adopting the standards to facilitate e-prescribing is one of the key action items in the government's plan to expedite the adoption of electronic medical records and build a national electronic health information infrastructure in the United States.

The MMA created a new voluntary prescription drug benefit under Medicare Part D. Although e-prescribing will be optional for physicians and pharmacies, Medicare Part D will require drug plans participating in the new prescription benefit to support electronic prescribing.

The benefits of eRx are many. The eRx speeds up the processing of renewing prescriptions and provides information about the formulary-based coverage for the patient. Designed to prevent medication errors, each prescription can be electronically checked for dosage, interactions with other prescriptions, and duplications. However, the costs of purchasing, maintaining, and educating staff may account for the low usage by providers. As of the writing of this text, there are no defined costs for the program. At present, it is voluntary. The Centers for Medicare and Medicaid Services (CMS) continues to attempt to improve the overall process. In late 2011, the CMS released new rules in an attempt to encourage more physicians to participate.

Although the use of eRx is low, many physicians now have the ability, through their EHR system, to have an electronically produced prescription completed for the patient. This helps cut down on errors due to poor handwriting. It also creates a record in the EHR.

Health Information Technology for Economic and Clinical Health Act (HITECH)

In response to the severe economic downturn in 2007–2009, Congress approved the **American Recovery and Reinvestment Act of 2009 (ARRA)**. The act was designed to pump federal stimulus funds into the economy to protect jobs in the private sector and to support spending programs at the state level in jeopardy from declining state revenues.

As part of ARRA, the **Health Information Technology for Economic and Clinical Health Act (HITECH)** was approved. The act serves the dual purpose of injecting stimulus funds into the economy and providing incentives for medical facilities to implement EHRs in the standardized format mandated under HIPAA.

In April 2018, CMS renamed the Meaningful Use incentive program as the Promoting Operability program. The change moved the focus of the program beyond the requirements of Meaningful Use to the interoperability of EHRs to improve data collection and submission, and patient access to health information.

Program implementation under the act was delegated to the CMS. Final regulations for the EHR program were released on July 13, 2010. Beginning in 2015, Medicare payment penalties were imposed on healthcare providers that had not implemented EHRs under the guidelines.

The final regulations from the CMS totaled 864 pages and established Stage 1 criteria for "meaningful use." The following Health Outcomes Policy Priorities were established:

- Improve quality, safety, efficiency, and reduce health disparities.
- Engage patients and families in their health care.
- Improve care coordination.
- Ensure adequate privacy and security protections for personal health information.

For each of these priorities, the final regulations define the professionals and healthcare facilities covered by the regulations and establish Stage 1 measurements for compliance.

EHR is a major change in the way healthcare organizations do business. Several studies have been completed that indicate that the costs for implementing an EHR either in the physician's office or the hospital are a major barrier.

In data from 2019 and 2021, 86 percent of non-Federal general acute care hospitals had adopted a 2015 Edition certified EHR. By contrast, only 40 percent of rehabilitation hospitals and 23 percent of specialty hospitals had adopted a 2015 Edition certified EHR.

Approximately 9 in 10 hospitals used their EHR data to inform clinical practice in 2017, according to a new report by the Department of Health and Human Services' Office of the National Coordinator for Health Information Technology, based on data from the AHA Annual Survey Information Technology Supplement. About 8 in 10 hospitals used their EHR data to support quality improvement, monitor patients' safety, or measure organization performance; 7 in 10 used them to identify high-risk patients, create individual provider profiles, measure unit performance, or inform strategic planning; 6 in 10 used them to identify care gaps for patients or assess adherence to guidelines; and 5 in 10 used them to develop an approach to query for data.

Knowledge Check 13.2

1. Why is the electronic health record (EHR) so important in providing quality patient care?

_____

_____

_____

2. Perform research on the costs to implement meaningful use EHR for a physician's office, for a dentist's office, and for a hospital setting.

_____

_____

_____

Coding and ICD-10-CM

For providers to be paid, they must submit bills to the appropriate payers. Payers must know what was done (the procedure) and why it was done (the diagnosis). Over the course of many years, the United States has developed a series of codes, both numeric and alphanumeric, to identify the procedure performed and why it was done.

The Healthcare Common Procedure Coding System (HCPCS) was developed originally by CMS for use when coding services provided to Medicare patients. It is now the federally mandated coding system for physician services. The services may be a simple office visit, the reading of an x-ray, or major surgery. Current procedural terminology (CPT) is used to identify physician and other provider care services. The system is unique to the United States. Other countries have their own physician service coding systems.

Coding diagnoses is a more complicated process. The United States, along with most other countries, uses the International Classification of Diseases (ICD). The origins of ICD date back to the 1850s when the International Statistical Institute created a classification system for causes of death worldwide. The World Health Organization (WHO) took over the responsibility for ICD in 1948 with the sixth edition. It was in the sixth edition that causes of morbidity were added. ICD is now the international standard diagnostic classification system for all morbidity and mortality. This standardization allows for analysis worldwide of the incidence and prevalence of disease.

The **International Classification of Diseases, Edition 10 (ICD-10-CM and ICD-10-PCS)** is the result of a world-wide initiative for the improvement of medical diagnosis codes. The ICD-10-CM is more specific in detail and should lead to improved accuracy in coding of diagnoses. The code set increased from some 13,000 codes to approximately 69,000 codes. Diagnostic codes moved from a possible five-digit numeric code to a seven-digit alphanumeric code.

ICD-10-CM does not include inpatient procedure codes. The United States contracted with 3M Health Information Systems to create **ICD-10-Procedure Coding System (ICD-10-PCS)**. This was done to provide a coding system for inpatient procedures for both statistical and billing purposes. A coding system was developed for ICD-9-PCS, but again the lack of specificity created problems. ICD-9-PCS had approximately 3,000 codes, while ICD-10-PCS has as many as 87,000 approved codes. ICD-10-PCS is unique to the United States. Figures 13-3 and 13-4 illustrate the differences between the ICD-9 system and the ICD-10 system.

The implementation of the EHR, along with the implementation of ICD-10, are major changes in the way the U.S. healthcare providers conduct their business. All providers of care, as well as insurance companies and other payers, are affected by these dramatic changes. Organizations must plan ahead and be prepared to make significant financial investment in these new technologies. Box 13-2 outlines the steps recommended by the CMS.

BOX 13-2 Recommended Steps for Implementation of ICD-10

- **Situational Analysis**
  - Identify stakeholders.
  - Assess impact.
  - Formulate strategies and identify goals.
  - Develop education/training plans for employees at all levels.

- Develop information systems/technology systems change implementation plan that includes testing and "go live" plans.
- Plan for documentation changes.
- **Strategic Implementation/Organizing**
  - Acquire resources to implement the plan.
  - Evaluate financial impact on organization.
- **Planning for Strategic Control**
  - Develop objectives.
  - Plan measurement tools.
  - Plan evaluation strategies.
  - Plan action steps for implementation.

Source: Centers for Medicare and Medicaid Services (CMS)

ICD-9-CM Diagnosis Codes	ICD-10-CM Diagnosis Codes
3–4 numbers in length	3–7 characters in length
Approximately 13,000 codes	Approximately 69,000 codes
Digit 1 may be alpha (E or V) or numeric; digits 2–5 are numeric.	Digit 1 is alpha, digits 2 and 3 are numeric, and digits 4–7 are alpha or numeric.
Limited space for adding new codes	Flexible for adding new codes
Lacks detail	Very specific
Lacks laterality	Has laterality
Difficult to analyze data due to nonspecific codes	Specificity improves coding accuracy and richness of data for analysis
Codes are nonspecific and do not adequately define diagnoses needed for medical research	Detail improves the accuracy of data used for medical research
Does not support interoperability, because it is not used by other countries	Supports interoperability and the exchange of health data between other countries and the United States
ICD-9-CM Procedure Codes	ICD-10-PCS Procedure Codes
3–4 numbers in length	7 alpha-numeric characters in length
Approximately 3,000 codes	Approximately 87,000 codes
Based on outdated technology	Reflects current usage of medical terminology and devices
Limited space for adding new codes	Flexible for adding new codes
Lacks detail	Very specific
Lacks laterality	Has laterality
Generic terms for body parts	Provides detailed descriptions of methodology and approach for procedures
Limits DRG assignment	Allows DRG definitions to better recognize new technologies and devices
Lacks precision to adequately define procedures	Precisely defines procedures with detail regarding body part, approach, any device used, and qualifying information

Figure 13-3 Comparison of ICD-9-CM and ICD-10-CM-PCS

ICD-9-CM	ICD-10-CM
Pressure ulcer codes	Pressure ulcer codes
9 location codes (707.00–707.09)	Shows more specific locations as well as depth 125 codes; example is: L89131 – Pressure ulcer of right lower back, stage I L89132 – Pressure ulcer of right lower back, stage II L89133 – Pressure ulcer of right lower back, stage III L89134 – Pressure ulcer of right lower back, stage IV
ICD-9-PCS	**ICD-10-PCS**
Angioplasty	Angioplasty
1 code 39.50	1,170 codes specifying body part, approach and device, including: 047K04Z dilation of right femoral artery with drug-eluting intraluminal device, open approach 047K0DZ dilation of right femoral artery with intraluminal device, open approach 047KOZZ dilation of right femoral artery, open approach

Figure 13-4 Examples of ICD-9-CM and ICD-10-CM

Key Concepts

- The adoption of various national laws has created new requirements for the entire healthcare industry.

- There is an expectation that healthcare providers ensure the privacy and security of the health record.

- ICD-10-CM and ICD-10-PCS are critical changes that must be implemented to provide for a better way to analyze healthcare trends in the United States and the world.

- Adopting health information technology is difficult due to the diverse interests of the providers, the payers, and the government.

References

Preface

Carbajol, E. (2022). *Number of Active Physicians by State*. Retrieved on June 6, 2022, from https://www.beckershospitalreview.com/rankings-and-ratings/number-of-active-physicians-by-state.html

Health Affairs. (2022). *National Health Expenditure Projections, 2021–30: Growth to Moderate as COVID-19 Impacts Wane*. Retrieved on June 6, 2022, from https://www.healthaffairs.org/doi/10.1377/hlthaff.2022.00113

Plescia, M. (2022). *Health Spending Grew 3.4% in 2021 Report Finds: 7 Things to Know*. Retrieved on June 6, 2022, from https://www.beckershospitalreview.com/finance/health-spending-grew-3-4-in-2021-report-finds-7-things-to-know.html

Section I

American Hospital Association. (2019). *AHA Annual Survey*. Retrieved on January 30, 2022, from https://www.aha.org/statistics/fast-facts-us-hospitals

American Hospital Association. (2021). *Fact Sheet: Strengthening the Healthcare Workforce*. Retrieved on February 20, 2022, from https://www.aha.org/fact-sheets/2021-05-26-fact-sheet-strengthening-health-care-workforce

Assistant Secretary for Planning and Evaluation (ASPE) (2020). *Medicare Beneficiaries Use of Telehealth in 2020: Trends by Beneficiary Characteristics and Location*. Retrieved on January 30, 2022, from https://aspe.hhs.gov/reports/medicare-beneficiary-use-telehealth-visits-early-data-start-covid-19-pandemic

Center on Budget and Policy Priorities. (2021). *Most of the Budget Goes Toward Defense, Social Security and Major Health Programs*. Retrieved on February 8, 2022, from https://www.cbpp.org/most-of-budget-goes-toward-defense-social-security-and-major-health-programs-2

Centers for Disease Control and Prevention. (2019). *Urgent Care Center and Retail Health Clinic Utilization Among Children: United States, 2019*. Retrieved on January 30, 2022, from https://www.cdc.gov/nchs/products/databriefs/db393.htm#fig1

Centers for Medicare & Medicaid Services. (2015). *Nursing Homes: Nursing Home Data Compendium*. Retrieved on January 30, 2022 from https://www.cms.gov/Medicare/Provider-Enrollment-and-Certification/CertificationandComplianc/NHs

Centers for Medicare & Medicaid Services. (2016). *CMS Statistics Reference booklet: Table 11.1 Inpatient hospitals/trends*. Retrieved on January 30, 2022, from https://www.cms.gov/Research-Statistics-Data-and-Systems/Statistics-Trends-and-Reports/CMS-Statistics-Reference-Booklet/2016

Centers for Medicare & Medicaid Services. (2019). *Design and development of the Diagnosis Related Group (DRG)*. Retrieved on January 30, 2022, from https://www.cms.gov/icd10m/version37-fullcode-cms/fullcode_cms/Design_and_development_of_the_Diagnosis_Related_Group_(DRGs).pdf

Centers for Medicare & Medicaid Services. (2021). *American Rescue Plan and the Marketplace Fact Sheet*. Retrieved on February 20, 2022, from https://www.cms.gov/newsroom/fact-sheets/american-rescue-plan-and-marketplace

Centers for Medicare & Medicaid Services. (2021). *New HHS Data Show More Americans than Ever Have Health Coverage through the Affordable Care Act, June 5, 2021*. Retrieved on February 8, 2022, from https://www.cms.gov/newsroom/press-releases/new-hhs-data-show-more-americans-ever-have-health-coverage-through-affordable-care-act

Congressional Budget Office. (2007). *The Long Term Budget Outlook*. Retrieved on February 8, 2022, from https://www.cbo.gov/publication/41650?index=8877

Congressional Budget Office. (2017). *Modify TRICARE enrollment Fees and Cost Sharing for Working-Age Military Retirees*. Retrieved on February 8, 2022, from https://www.cbo.gov/budget-options/2018/54763

Department of Health and Human Services. (2019). *The Department of Justice Healthcare Fraud and Abuse Control Program Annual Report for Fiscal Year 2019*. Retrieved on February 20, 2022, from https://oig.hhs.gov/publications/docs/hcfac/FY2019-hcfac.pdf

Health Affairs. (2020). *National Health Cares Spending in 2020: Growth Driven by Federal Spending in Response to The COVID 19 Pandemic*. Retrieved on January 30, 2022, from https://www.healthaffairs.org/doi/abs/10.1377/hlthaff.2021.01763

HealthCare.gov. (2022). *What's considered a High Deductible Health Plan?* Retrieved on February 8, 2022, from https://www.healthcare.gov/high-deductible-health-plan/

Kaiser Family Foundation. (2021). *KFF 2021 Employee Health Benefits Survey*. Retrieved on February 8, 2022, from https://www.kff.org/report-section/ehbs-2021-section-1-cost-of-health-insurance/

Office of the Assistant Secretary for Planning and Evaluation. (2021). *Access to Marketplace Plans with Low Premiums: Current Enrollees and the American Rescue Plan.* Retrieved on February 20, 2022, from https://aspe.hhs.gov/reports/access-marketplace-plans-low-premiums-current-enrollees-american-rescue-plan

U.S. Census Bureau. (2020). *2020 Census Will Help Policymakers Prepare for the Incoming Wave of Aging Boomers.* Retrieved on February 20, 2022, from https://www.census.gov/library/stories/2019/12/by-2030-all-baby-boomers-will-be-age-65-or-older.html

U.S. Department of Health & Human Services. (2020). *HHS FY 2022 Budget in Brief.* Retrieved on February 8, 2022, from https://www.hhs.gov/about/budget/fy2022/index.html

U.S. Department of Labor. (2021). *An Employee's Guide to Health Benefits Under COBRA-US.* Retrieved on February 8, 2022, from https://www.dol.gov/agencies/ebsa/laws-and-regulations/laws/cobra

World Health Organization. (2019). *Who Calls for Urgent Action to reduce Patient Harm in Healthcare?* Retrieved on February 20, 2022, from https://www.who.int/news/item/13-09-2019-who-calls-for-urgent-action-to-reduce-patient-harm-in-healthcare

Section II

Centers for Medicare and Medicaid Services. (2016). *CMS Roadmaps*. Retrieved on January 23, 2022, from https://www.cms.gov/medicare/quality-initiatives-patient-assessment-instruments/qualityinitiativesgeninfo/downloads/roadmapoverview_oea_1-16.pdf

Fernando, J. (2021). *Current Ratio*. Retrieved on April 7, 2022, from https://www.investopedia.com/terms/c/currentratio.asp

Fischer, M. J. (2000). Luca Pacioli on business profits. Journal of Business Ethics, *25*(4), 299-312. https://doi-org.libauth.purdueglobal.edu/10.1023/A:1006281415873

Internal Revenue Service. (2022). *Publication 946 (2020), How To Depreciate Property*. Retrieved on January 23, 2022, from https://www.irs.gov/publications/p946

Office of Financial Management. (2022). *State Administrative and Accounting Manual*. Retrieved on March 20, 2022, from https://ofm.wa.gov/accounting/saam/glossary

Seth, S. (2021). *Quick Ratio*. Retrieved on April, 7, 2022, from https://www.investopedia.com/terms/q/quickratio.asp#toc-quick-ratio-vs-current-ratio

United States Census Bureau. (2017). *Debt for Households, by Type of Debt and Selected Characteristics*. Retrieved on January 23, 2022, from https://www.census.gov/data/tables/2017/demo/wealth/wealth-asset-ownership.html

Section III

American Hospital Association. (2019). ONC: *Nearly All Hospitals Use EHR data to Inform Clinical Practice.* Retrieved on May 29, 2022, from https://www.aha.org/news/headline/2019-04-17-onc-nearly-all-hospitals-use-ehr-data-inform-clinical-practice

Beckers Hospital CFO Report. (2022). *Mass General Brigham posts $867M quarterly net loss.* Retrieved from https://www.beckershospitalreview.com/finance/mass-general-brigham-posts-867m-quarterly-net-loss.html?utm_campaign=bhr&utm_source=website&utm_content=latestarticles

Beckers Hospital CFO Report. (2022). *7 Recent Hospital, Health System Credit Rating Actions*. Retrieved on May 15, 2022, from https://www.beckershospitalreview.com/finance/7-recent-hospital-health-system-credit-rating-actions.html

Carlson, R. (2020). *How to Set Up and Manage a Petty Cash Account?* Retrieved April 20, 2022, from https://www.thebalancesmb.com/managing-a-small-business-petty-cash-account-393001

Centers for Medicare & Medicaid Services. (2022). *Are You a Covered Entity?* Retrieved on May 21, 2022, from https://www.cms.gov/Regulations-and-Guidance/Administrative-Simplification/HIPAA-ACA/AreYouaCoveredEntity

Centers for Medicare and Medicaid Services. (2021). *ICD-10 Final Rule*. Retrieved on May 28, 2022, from https://www.cms.gov/Medicare/Coding/ICD10

Dressner, M. (2017). *Hospital Workers: An Assessment of Occupational Injuries and Illnesses*. Retrieved on May 22, 2022, from https://www.bls.gov/opub/mlr/2017/article/hospital-workers-an-assessment-of-occupational-injuries-and-illnesses.htm

Federal Deposit Insurance Corporation. (2021). *Bank Failures in Brief – Summary 2001 through 2022*. Retrieved on May 15, 2022, from https://www.fdic.gov/bank/historical/bank/

FindLaw. (2020). *What are Intentional Torts?* Retrieved on May 22, 2022, from https://www.findlaw.com/injury/torts-and-personal-injuries/what-are-intentional-torts.html

FINRA. (2022). *Agency Securities*. Retrieved on May 15, 2022, from https://www.finra.org/investors/learn-to-invest/types-investments/bonds/types-of-bonds/agency-securities

Foresight. (2020). *2021 Workers Comp Statistics that Reveal Key Focus Areas*. Retrieved on May 22, 2022, from https://getforesight.com/workers-compensation-statistics/

Hayhurst, C. (2018). *To Retain New Patients, Give Them an Appointment Stat*. Retrieved on May 20, 2022, from https://www.athenahealth.com/knowledge-hub/financial-performance/retain-new-patients-give-them-appointment-stat

HIPAA Journal. (2022). *2021–2022 HIPAA violation Cases and Penalties*. Retrieved on May 28, 2022, from https://www.hipaajournal.com/2020-hipaa-violation-cases-and-penalties/

HIPAA Journal. (2022). *HIPAA Violations*. Retrieved on May 28, 2022, from https://www.hipaajournal.com/hipaa-violation-cases/

National Library of Medicine. (2020). *Evaluating the Impact of Patient No-shows on Service Quality*. Retrieved from https://www.ncbi.nlm.nih.gov/pmc/articles/PMC7280239/

Norris, J. (2020). *Determine Your Break-Even Point*. Retrieved on April 12, 2022, from https://www.physicianspractice.com/view/determine-your-break-even-point

Office of the National Coordinator for Health Information Technology. (2022). *Adoption of Electronic Health Records by Hospital Service Type 2019-2021*. Retrieved on May 29, 2022, from https://www.healthit.gov/data/quickstats/adoption-electronic-health-records-hospital-service-type-2019-2021

Rundio, A. (2019). *Budget Development for Nurse Managers*. Retrieved on April 12, 2022, from https://nursingcentered.sigmanursing.org/features/top-stories/budget-development-for-the-nurse-manager

United States Department of Labor. (2019). *Worker Safety in Hospitals*. Retrieved on May 22, 2022, from https://www.osha.gov/hospitals

Glossary

A

Accounting   Accounting is a process, and the end product from this process is financial information.

Accounting equation   An accounting equation is the equation used regularly in the accounting field in double-entry accounting. The equation can be written in several different ways, such as Assets = Liabilities + Net worth or Net worth = Assets − Liabilities.

Accounts payable   Accounts payable is the amount owed by the medical facility for goods and services purchased on credit.

Accounts receivable   Accounts receivable is the cumulative balance of all of the individual charges for medical services due from patients and insurance companies not paid in cash at time of service.

Accrual accounting   is the system of accounting that records revenues in the accounting period in which they are earned and expenses in the accounting period in which the resources are used.

Accumulated depreciation   Accumulated depreciation is the total value of the annual charges for **depreciation** (see later definition) of an asset since that asset was placed into service.

Affirmative action   Affirmative action is the process of developing procedures to ensure that individuals in protected classes (defined later in this list) have equal access to employment.

Age Discrimination in Employment Act (ADEA) of 1967   Age Discrimination in Employment Act (ADEA) of 1967 requires that workers over the age of 40 receive equal treatment in the workplace.

American Recovery and Reinvestment Act of 2009 (ARRA)   The American Recovery and Reinvestment Act of 2009 (ARRA) was approved as a stimulus for capital investment. The act included funding for computerized medical records in a standardized format.

American Rescue Plan Act of 2021   American Rescue Plan Act of 2021 provides additional relief to address the continued impact of COVID-19 (i.e., coronavirus disease 2019) on the economy, public health, state and local governments, individuals, and businesses.

Americans with Disabilities Act (ADA) of 1990   Americans with Disabilities Act (ADA) of 1990 protects the rights of people who are disabled in the workplace and requires "reasonable accommodation" for people with disabilities.

Annual budget   The annual budget of the organization combines the annual revenue budget and the annual expenditure budget.

Assets   Assets are the items of financial value owned by the medical facility.

Automobile liability insurance   Automobile liability insurance protects against risk from loss in accidents involving vehicles owned by the business.

B

Baby boomers   Baby boomers are members of the generation born between 1946 and 1964.

Balance billing   Balance billing is the prohibited practice of billing patients for amounts greater than contract rates for medical services.

Balance sheet   The balance sheet displays all the items owned by the business, all debts that are owed, and the book value of the business at a certain point in time.

Balanced Budget Act of 1997   Balanced Budget Act of 1997 authorized Medicare Advantage plans as an alternative to traditional Medicare.

Balloon maturity   Balloon maturity is an exceptionally large single payment due at a fixed date in the future.

Bank reconciliation   Bank reconciliation is the process of ensuring that the accounting records for the checking account agree with the monthly bank statement.

Bonds   Bonds are securities (see term later in this list) where the issuer borrows money from an investor and promises to repay the investor a fixed principal and interest at a stated rate on a specific date.

Book value   The book value of an asset is the value asset on the financial statements representing the original cost of the asset less the accumulated depreciation recorded since the asset was placed in use.

Bottom-up budgeting   Bottom-up budgeting is a participatory philosophy of budgeting, relying on unit managers to provide information on the unit's operational needs.

Break-even analysis   Break-even analysis is the budget mechanism that allows for the determination of the number of units of service that need to be provided to cover the organization's costs.

Budget   The budget is management's plan for a future period of time, expressed in dollars.

Budget amendment   A budget amendment is the official approval to move funds from one budget line item to another.

Budget control   Budget control is the level of flexibility provided to unit managers in using budgeted funds during the year.

Build Back Better Plan   Build Back Better Plan provides funding, establishes programs, and otherwise modifies provisions relating to a broad array of areas, including education, labor, child care, health care, taxes, immigration, and the environment.

C

Capital assets   Capital assets are items of higher than minimal value owned by the business, such as buildings and equipment, which have a relatively long, useful life.

Capital budget   The capital budget accounts for the major capital expenditures of the organization and is normally prepared to cover several budget years.

Capital expenses   Capital expenses are the annual costs related to the decline in value over time of assets with a relatively long, useful life.

Capitation plans   Capitation plans are insurance programs that pay providers a specific amount in advance to provide healthcare services to members. Providers are normally paid on a per-member, per-month (PMPM) basis. Unless otherwise stipulated in the contract, the provider bears the full costs of providing agreed services to members and accepts the monthly payment amounts as the full amount due under the contract.

Cash accounting   Cash accounting is the system of accounting that records revenues in the accounting period in which cash payment is received and expenses in the accounting period when payment is made.

Cash and cash equivalents   Cash and cash equivalents on the balance sheet combines cash, checking account balances, and short-term liquid investments such as certificates of deposit or treasury bills.

Cash budget   The cash budget projects revenues, expenditures, and cash flow on a monthly basis.

Cash drawer   The cash drawer, generally part of a cash register linked to the financial management system, is used to make change for patients paying cash for services provided.

Certificate of Need (CON)   A Certificate of Need (CON) is a legal document required in 36 states and federal jurisdictions issued by healthcare authorities prior to the expansion of an existing hospital or construction of a new facility.

Chart of accounts   The chart of accounts is the listing of all line items used in the budget and accounting system to identify specific revenues and expenditures.

Children's Health Insurance Program (CHIP) of 1997   Children's Health Insurance Program (CHIP) of 1997 expanded Medicaid to include children in families earning above the poverty level.

Clinton Health Care Plan of 1993   The Clinton Health Care Plan of 1993 was the failed attempt to secure universal healthcare coverage for all Americans.

Consistency   Consistency is the accounting policy requiring that once the proper accounting treatment for an issue has been determined, the same process should be applied for years.

Consolidated Omnibus Budget Reconciliation Act (COBRA)   Consolidated Omnibus Budget Reconciliation Act (COBRA) provides continuation of group health insurance benefits when an individual is separated from the employer because of termination of employment, divorce from a covered employee, or the death of the employee.

Contra account   A contra account is used to reduce the value of an asset account by the estimated loss in value of the asset. Contra accounts are most commonly used to record the estimated value of uncollectible accounts receivable and to record accumulated depreciation of capital assets.

Corporation   A corporation is a business entity where the business is separate and distinct from its ownership, providing limited liability to its stockholders.

Credit risk   Credit risk is the danger that the value of a security held will fall with declines in the financial strength of the company issuing the security.

Credits   Credits in double-entry accounting are used to post increases in revenue, liability, and equity accounts and to post decreases in asset and expense accounts.

Crime insurance   Crime insurance protects against risks from loss of money and securities, such as employee embezzlement.

Current assets   Current assets are those assets that will be used by the business within a 12-month period.

Current liabilities   Current liabilities are amounts owed by a business that are expected to be paid during the next 12 months.

Current ratio   Current ratio compares the balance sheet value of current assets to current liabilities.

D

Debits   Debits in double-entry accounting are used to post increases in asset and expense accounts and to post decreases in revenue, liability, and equity accounts.

Debt-to-net-worth ratio   Debt-to-net-worth ratio compares the debt (liabilities owed) of the business to net worth.

Depreciation expense   Depreciation expense is the measurement of loss in value of a capital asset, charged annually, as it ages or is used up during business.

Directors and officers (D&O) insurance   Directors and officers (D&O) insurance protects against risks involving actions of directors and officers of the business.

Double-entry accounting   Double-entry accounting requires that every individual entry into the financial system include one or more debits balanced and offset by one or more credits.

E

Electronic health record (EHR)   An electronic health record (EHR) is the health record of a patient kept in an electronic format by providers of medical service.

Electronic prescriptions (eRx)   Electronic prescriptions (eRx) are an initiative of the federal government to have physicians use electronic means to send prescriptions to the patient and pharmacies.

Encounters   Encounters are the number of units of patient care provided by the medical facility.

Equal Employment Opportunity Commission (EEOC)   Equal Employment Opportunity Commission (EEOC) was created by Title VII of the Civil Rights Act of 1964 to enforce actions on discrimination in the hiring process.

Equal Pay Act of 1963   Equal Pay Act of 1963 established the standard that similar wages must be paid for similar work.

Equity   Equity is ownership.

Equity ownership,   Equity ownership, also known as net worth, is the book value of the business for the owner, partner, or shareholders.

Expenditure budget   Expenditure budget is the combination of approved operating budgets for the various departments, current year approved capital replacements and improvements, and cost items.

Expenses   Expenses serve as a measurement of the resources used, such as personnel and supplies, to generate revenues.

F

Fair Labor Standards Act (FLSA) of 1938   Fair Labor Standards Act (FLSA) of 1938 establishes minimum wage rates and regulates the requirement for overtime pay.

Family and Medical Leave Act (FMLA) of 1993   Family and Medical Leave Act (FMLA) of 1993 provides a guarantee of continuation of employment after up to 12 weeks away from the job for family or medical issues.

Federal Deposit Insurance Corporation (FDIC)   Federal Deposit Insurance Corporation (FDIC) is the federal agency insuring bank deposits for individual investors.

Fee-for-service   Fee-for-service is the reimbursement to a medical service provider for specified services based on a fee schedule established by the third-party payer and agreed to by the provider.

Financial accounting   Financial accounting is involved in the preparation of financial documents that are primarily intended for outside users.

Fiscal year   Fiscal year is a consecutive 12-month period chosen by the business to report financial operations.

Fixed rate   Fixed rate on a loan or security denotes that the interest rate will remain constant or change only on a predetermined schedule.

Float   Float refers to the length of time from the date a check is written until the check clears the issuing bank and funds are withdrawn from the issuer's account.

Foreign exchange risk   Foreign exchange risk is the danger in investing in foreign securities that the value of a security will be worth less in U.S. dollars if the currency exchange rate changes.

Full disclosure   Full disclosure is the principle that any events that may have an impact on the financial condition of the organization need to be disclosed in the annual financial report.

Full-time equivalent (FTE)   A full-time equivalent (FTE) position is based on one employee working 8 hours per day, 5 days per week, for 52 weeks per year.

G

General ledger   A general ledger is the journal of original entry records for each day of events. This is shown as the date the transaction occurred.

General liability insurance   General liability insurance protects against risks from common occurrences such as slip and fall.

Generally accepted accounting principles (GAAP)   Generally accepted accounting principles (GAAP) are the basic standards and rules that accountants follow in recording financial transactions and reporting results.

Going concern concept   Going concern concept is the accounting principle that values assets and liabilities of the business under the assumption that the medical facility will continue in business, with receivables being collected when due and payables paid from revenues of continuing business operations.

Goodwill   Goodwill is a business asset recognized when a business is purchased for an amount greater than the total book value of the assets purchased.

Government policy risk   Government policy risk is the danger that the value of a security will fall based on changes in policy by the government in the country where the security is issued.

Gross domestic product (GDP)   Gross domestic product (GDP) is the total economic output of the goods and services produced within the borders of the country, regardless of the nationality of the companies producing the goods or services.

Gross medical service revenues   Gross medical service revenues are what the medical facility would have received if all services provided were billed and paid at the full price charged to private-pay patients.

Gross national product (GNP)   Gross national product (GNP) measures the total output of all the business enterprises of a country, whether produced within or outside of the borders of the country.

Gross pay   Gross pay is the amount of the employee's periodic paycheck before taxes and other deductions.

H

Health information technology (HIT)   Health information technology (HIT) is the hardware, software, integrated technologies or related licenses, intellectual property, upgrades, or packaged solutions sold as services that are maintenance, access, or exchange of health information.

Health Information Technology for Economic and Clinical Health Act (HITECH)   Health Information Technology for Economic and Clinical Health Act (HITECH) of 2009 provided federal stimulus funding for the automation of healthcare records.

Health Insurance Portability and Accountability Act of 1996 (HIPAA)   Health Insurance Portability and Accountability Act of 1996 (HIPAA) provides for the portability of healthcare benefits between employers, ensures the privacy of healthcare information, and requires the standardization of electronic healthcare communications.

Health maintenance organizations (HMOs)   Health maintenance organizations (HMOs) are a form of managed care healthcare insurance. A primary care physician "gatekeeper" coordinates patient care and directs patients to specialists. Plan participants are required to use medical service providers within the HMO network.

Hospice care   Hospice care is designed to meet the needs of dying patients and their families, keeping the patient free of pain and attending to the spiritual and emotional issues faced during this stage of life.

Hospital Survey and Construction Act of 1946   The Hospital Survey and Construction Act of 1946 required the states to implement plans for hospital construction programs and provided federal grants to finance the construction of community hospitals.

I

Income statement   The income statement reports revenues, expenses, and net income over the period of time covered in the report.

Incremental budgeting   Incremental budgeting starts with the current approved budget and adds funds for inflation and projected demands for service.

Inflation   Inflation is the increase over time of the general level of costs of goods and services in the economy.

Inpatient facilities   Inpatient facilities, most commonly hospitals, provide medical services where the patient resides in the facility for a minimum of one overnight stay.

Insurance   Insurance protects businesses, individuals, or groups from the risks of financial loss. Premium payments for the transfer of risk are pooled with a large group of participants.

Insurance contracts   Insurance contracts are legal agreements between the medical facility and an insurance company, detailing the terms of the agreement and specifying reimbursement rates for medical services.

Intangible assets   Intangible assets are assets of value to the business, but do not have a physical existence, such as patents, copyrights, goodwill, and investment in research and development.

Interest   Interest is the cost incurred to borrow money or the payment received to loan or invest money.

Interest rate risk   Interest rate risk is the danger that the value of a security will fall if market interest rates increase.

International Classification of Diseases, Edition 10 (ICD-10-CM and ICD-10-PCS)   The International Classification of Diseases, Edition 10 (ICD-10-CM and ICD-10-PCS) is a worldwide initiative for the improvement of medical diagnosis codes.

Issuer   Issuer in a bond offering is the legal entity borrowing the funds and agreeing to repayment terms.

L

Liabilities   Liabilities are what are owed by the medical facility for unpaid bills for goods and services and longer-term debt, such as balances on bank and equipment loans.

Lilly Ledbetter Fair Pay Act of 2009   Lilly Ledbetter Fair Pay Act of 2009 amended the filing deadlines under Title VII of the Civil Rights Act of 1964.

Limited liability partnership (LLP)   A limited liability partnership (LLP) is a structure authorized under state statutes for a medical services partnership to limit the partners' liability in malpractice.

Line of credit   Line of credit is an agreement allowing for draw up to a maximum amount in a certain period of time.

Litigation   Litigation is the process of taking a legal proceeding through the courts.

London Interbank Offered Rate (LIBOR)   London Interbank Offered Rate (LIBOR) is an accepted standard as a benchmark for variable rate loans and investments.

Long-term-care facilities   Long-term-care facilities, such as nursing homes and life-care facilities, meet extended care needs of patients who are no longer able to live independently.

M

Managed care   Managed care is a term used to describe efforts to provide quality care at a reasonable cost.

Managerial accounting   Managerial accounting is involved in the preparation of financial documents that are primarily intended for internal use within the organization.

Massachusetts Health Care Reform Law of 2006   The Massachusetts Health Care Reform Law of 2006 was state legislation providing universal healthcare coverage for all citizens of the state of Massachusetts.

Matching   Matching is the accounting principle that states that revenues are posted in the accounting period when services are provided and expenses are posted when resources are used.

Materiality   Materiality is the accounting principle that requires that any accounting error that will have a significant impact on the financial statements of the business entity must be corrected.

Medicaid   Medicaid was approved in the Social Security Amendments of 1965 to provide healthcare coverage for low-income Americans.

Medical facility average cost   Medical facility average cost is the total operating costs of the practice divided by the number of patient visits.

Medical facility marginal cost   Medical facility marginal cost is the added cost to provide medical services for one additional patient visit.

Medical malpractice insurance   Medical malpractice insurance protects against risks of loss from the actions of medical professionals.

Medicare   Medicare was approved in the Social Security Amendments of 1965 to provide healthcare coverage for Americans 65 and older and those with certain disabilities.

Medicare Improvements for Patients and Providers Act (MIPPA)   The Medicare Improvements for Patients and Providers Act (MIPPA) provides funding to agencies and organizations in all states or Native American tribes that are used for financial assistance to help eligible Medicare beneficiaries reduce their premiums and deductibles.

Medicare Modernization Act (MMA)   The Medicare Modernization Act (MMA) helped establish prescription drug coverage. It is viewed as a large benefit in Medicare history.

Medicare Prescription Drug, Improvement, and Modernization Act of 2003 (MMA)   Medicare Prescription Drug, Improvement, and Modernization Act of 2003 (MMA) authorized Medicare Part D for prescription drug coverage for seniors.

N

Net income   Net income is the excess of revenues over expenses for the period of time accounted for in the income statement.

Net medical service revenue   Net medical service revenue is the amount of revenue expected to be received by the medical facility for services provided.

Net pay   Net pay is the actual amount of the employee's periodic paycheck.

Net worth   Net worth is the difference between total assets and total liabilities. Depending on the legal structure, terms used for net worth include owner's equity, capital stock and retained earnings, net assets, and fund balance.

Non-current assets   Non-current assets are those assets that will be used by the business for a period greater than 1 year.

Non-current liabilities   Non-current liabilities are amounts owed by a business that are expected to be paid at a date in the future more than 12 months away.

O

Occupational Safety and Health Administration (OSHA)   Occupational Safety and Health Administration (OSHA) is the federal agency that provides protections for employee safety in the workplace.

Operating budget   Operating budget, also commonly called the annual budget, combines the annual revenue budget and the annual expenditure budget.

Operating expenses   Operating expenses are the costs involved in running the business on a daily basis.

Oregon Health Plan   The Oregon Health Plan was the first attempt by a state government to implement universal health care.

Outpatient facilities   Outpatient facilities provide medical services without overnight stays.

P

Palliative care   Palliative care is the medical care provided to a patient at the last stages of life, designed to manage the symptoms of the patient's final illness and provide relief from pain.

Par value   Par value is the original stated price, or face amount, of the investment or bond.

Partnership   A partnership is a business owned by two or more individuals or entities.

Patient Protection and Affordable Care Act of 2010 (PPACA)   The Patient Protection and Affordable Care Act of 2010 (PPACA) is landmark healthcare reform, requiring most Americans to purchase healthcare insurance and expanding coverage requirements of existing group health insurance plans.

Petty cash fund   The petty cash fund of a business is used to account for small cash expenditures.

Practice management systems (PMS)   Practice management systems (PMS) are comprehensive computer software programs designed specifically for medical offices.

Precertification   Precertification is the requirement that the insurance company agree to the medical procedure in advance of service.

Preferred provider   Preferred provider healthcare insurance programs restrict plan participants to an approved list of providers who have contractually agreed to accept established reimbursement schedules for medical services.

Preferred provider organization (PPO) plans   Preferred provider organization (PPO) plans are a form of managed care. Under these types of plans, the third-party payer, normally an insurance company, will negotiate discounted fee schedules with primary care physicians, specialists, and hospitals.

Pregnancy Discrimination Act (PDA) of 1978   Pregnancy Discrimination Act (PDA) of 1978 requires that pregnancy be treated the same as any other medical or personal leave.

Private-pay patients   Private-pay patients are those patients who are responsible for the full financial costs of their medical care.

Professional corporation (PC)   A professional corporation (PC), also known as a professional association (PA), is a legal form of business established to allow proprietorships (defined below) to limit the liability of the owner.

Property insurance   Property insurance protects against risks to property owned by the business from exposures such as fire and natural disasters.

Proprietorship   A proprietorship is a business owned by one individual.

Protected classes   Protected classes are members of recognized minorities, women, individuals over age 40, disabled persons, and individuals with special religious beliefs.

Q

Quality management (QM)   Quality management (QM) is the growing profession dedicated to excellence in service delivery.

Quick ratio   Quick ratio is the current assets of cash, short-term investments, and accounts receivable compared to current liabilities.

R

Recovery Audit Contractor (RAC) Program   The Recovery Audit Contractor (RAC) Program is as public-private partnership designed to uncover improper payments in the Medicare and Medicaid programs.

Revenue budget   The revenue budget starts with the projected revenues from patient care, based on the statistical budget (see the following term), and adds nonpatient revenues to project total revenues for the budget year.

Revenue cycle management   Revenue cycle management deals with the collection of the full amount of funds owed for medical services as quickly and efficiently as possible.

Revenues   Revenues are the amounts earned by the medical facility in providing services to patients and clients.

Risk management   Risk management is the organized process to identify, evaluate, reduce or eliminate, and transfer to others the costs of risks to patients, visitors, and the organization's staff and assets.

Rule of 72   The Rule of 72 is an easy method to determine the number of years required for an investment to double in value at fixed annual rates of interest.

S

Salvage value   Salvage value is an accounting term referring to the amount of money expected to be realized from the sale of used assets, normally furniture and equipment.

Security   A security is a financial instrument that represents either financial ownership (corporate stocks) or a debt agreement (bonds or banking agreements with an interest rate and a fixed maturity date).

Severability clause   A severability clause is included in legislation and states that if any one section of the law is later ruled illegal, the balance of the law remains in full force and effect.

Sexual discrimination   Sexual discrimination is covered under The U.S. Equal Employment Opportunity Commission's (EEOC) extended Title VII of the Civil Rights Act of 1964 prohibiting discrimination on the basis of sexual orientation and gender identity. Sexual discrimination under Title VII also covers discrimination based on pregnancy, childbirth, or a related medical condition. This protection extends to prevent the employer from determining when the employee should take time off based on their pregnancy.

Sexual harassment   Sexual harassment results from unwelcome sexual advances, physical contact that creates a hostile environment, or requests for sexual favors.

Single payment loan   Single payment loan is a bank loan for a specific period of time with one payment at maturity.

Social Security Act of 1935   Social Security Act of 1935 provides income to retired and disabled workers, and their survivors, meeting eligibility requirements.

Social Security Amendments of 1965   Social Security Amendments of 1965 authorized the government programs of Medicare and Medicaid.

Spend-down   Spend-down is the term used for the process that occurs when an individual's financial resources are exhausted and the individual becomes eligible for Medicaid assistance in meeting nursing home bills.

Stakeholders   Stakeholders in health care include all people and outside organizations that are directly impacted by the performance of healthcare facilities.

Stale-dated checks   Stale-dated checks are checks issued by a business that have not been presented for payment within a reasonable period of time.

Statement of cash flows   The statement of cash flows supplements the balance sheet and income statement, providing the reader with information on the sources and uses of cash in the business.

Statistical budget   The statistical budget projects patient care revenues based on units of service to be provided and established reimbursement rates.

Straight-line method   Straight-line method is a method used to calculate accumulated depreciation. The formula is: (Purchase Price − Salvage Value/Years in Useful Life).

Subsequent events   Subsequent events are actions of a material nature, occurring after the end of the financial reporting period but prior to the date of the accountant's report, that need to be disclosed in the annual financial report.

T

Tangible assets   Tangible assets are those assets owned by the business, such as buildings and equipment, that have a physical existence.

Tax Equity and Fiscal Responsibility Act of 1982 (TEFRA)   The Tax Equity and Fiscal Responsibility Act of 1982 (TEFRA) abolished the former cost-plus Medicare reimbursement system and replaced it with standardized reimbursement tables.

Telehealth services   Telehealth services allow a patient to schedule an appointment and meet with a healthcare professional remotely. The healthcare professional assesses a patient's needs virtually. Usually, the appointment is through video or audio. Due to the national COVID-19 pandemic, telehealth appointments increased.

Term loan   Term loan is a bank loan over an extended period of time with required periodic payments.

The American Recovery and Reinvestment Act (ARRA) of 2009   The American Recovery and Reinvestment Act (ARRA) of 2009 was approved as a stimulus for capital investment. The act included funding for computerized medical records in a standardized format.

Time value of money   The time value of money is the concept of interest that a dollar available today is worth more than a dollar received in the future.

Title VII, Civil Rights Act of 1964   Title VII, Civil Rights Act of 1964 was the first major piece of legislation to prohibit discrimination in the hiring process.

Top-down budgeting   Top-down budgeting places the control for the development of the budget in the hands of a limited number of individuals at the top management level of the organization.

Tort   A tort is a civil legal action arising from a wrongful act that results in the injury to someone's person, reputation, or property.

Tort reform   Tort reform is the process to contain medical malpractice costs and is designed to place limits on non-economic and punitive damages, limit attorney fees, and shorten the statute of limitations for filing legal claims.

Trial balance   A trial balance is a listing of the current balances of all accounts in the financial system at a certain point in time to ensure that the total of the accounts with a debit balance equals the total of the accounts with a credit balance.

TRICARE insurance   TRICARE insurance provides healthcare insurance benefits for active members of the U.S. Armed Forces, retired military and National Guard and Reserve members, and their dependents.

V

Variable rate   Variable rate on a loan or security means that the interest rate will adjust periodically based on an index.

Variance analysis   Variance analysis is the periodic review of actual expenditures against the approved budget to determine compliance.

W

Workers' compensation insurance   Workers' compensation insurance provides medical treatment and continuation of income for employees injured on the job.

Z

Zero-base budgeting (ZBB)   Zero-base budgeting (ZBB) requires that each unit manager responsible for a budget justify every item in the budget from a base of zero each budget year.

Index